Basic Concept & Vocabulary Round-Up

948 Fun Reproducible Pictures & Auditory Bombardment Lists for Language Development

Written by
Beverly Foster
Illustrated by
Patti Rishforth

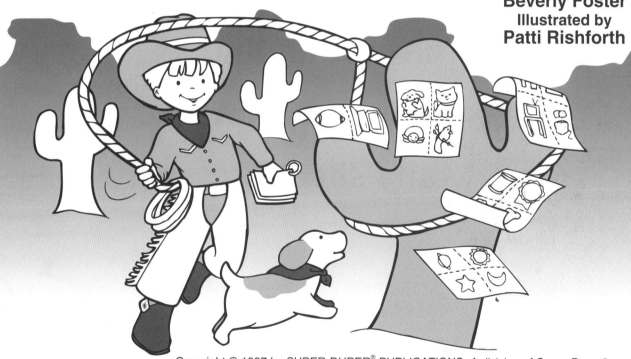

www.superduperinc.com
Post Office Box 24997, Greenville, SC 29616 USA
Call Toll Free 1-800-277-8737 • Fax 1-800-978-7379

ISBN# 1-58650-061-9

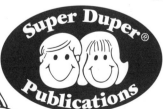

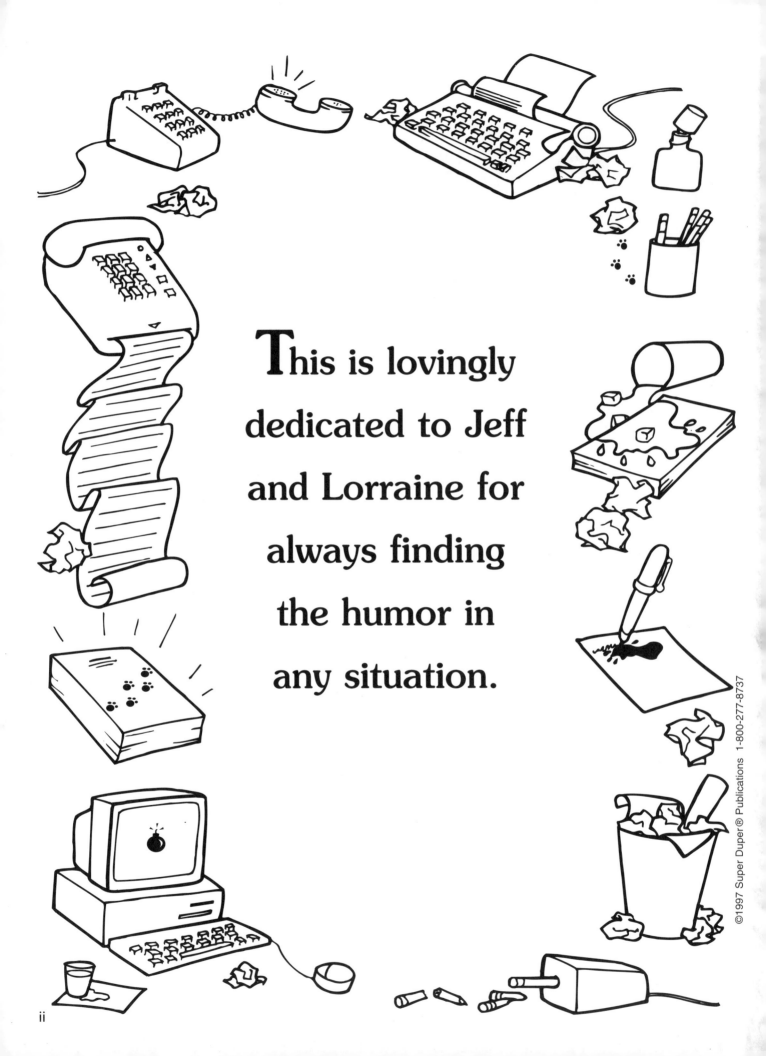

This is lovingly dedicated to Jeff and Lorraine for always finding the humor in any situation.

About the Author

Beverly Foster has earned a Masters Degree in Communication Disorders from the University of the Pacific in Stockton, California. In addition, she has received her Certificate of Clinical Competence in Speech-Language Pathology from the American Speech-Language-Hearing Association as well as her California State license. Currently, she is employed as a public school speech pathologist in the Elk Grove Unified School District. Ms. Foster has devoted much of her time in the designing and implementing of an innovative district-wide phonological program. Beverly resides in Elk Grove, California with her two children. Her hobbies include exercising, reading, calligraphy, cake decorating and traveling.

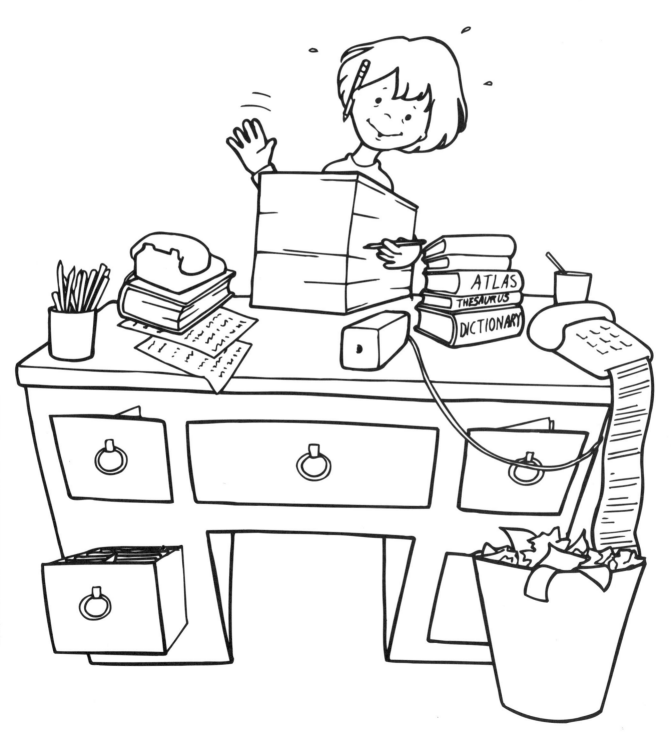

Table of Contents

I. Vocabulary Section

Animals/Pets

Occupations/Jobs

©1997 Super Duper® Publications 1-800-277-8737

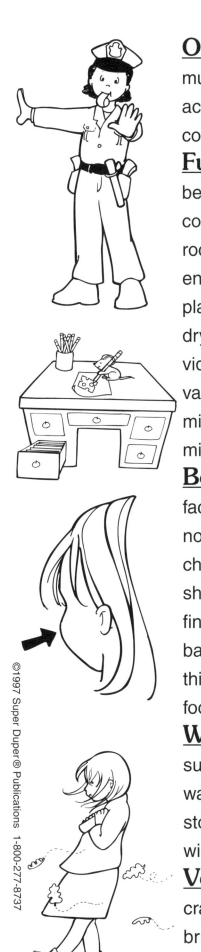

Occupations/Jobs (continued)

Furniture, Appliances and Accessories

Body Parts

Weather Words

Verbs

©1997 Super Duper® Publications 1-800-277-8737

Verbs (continued)

Tools

Sports

Kitchen Items and Eating Utensils

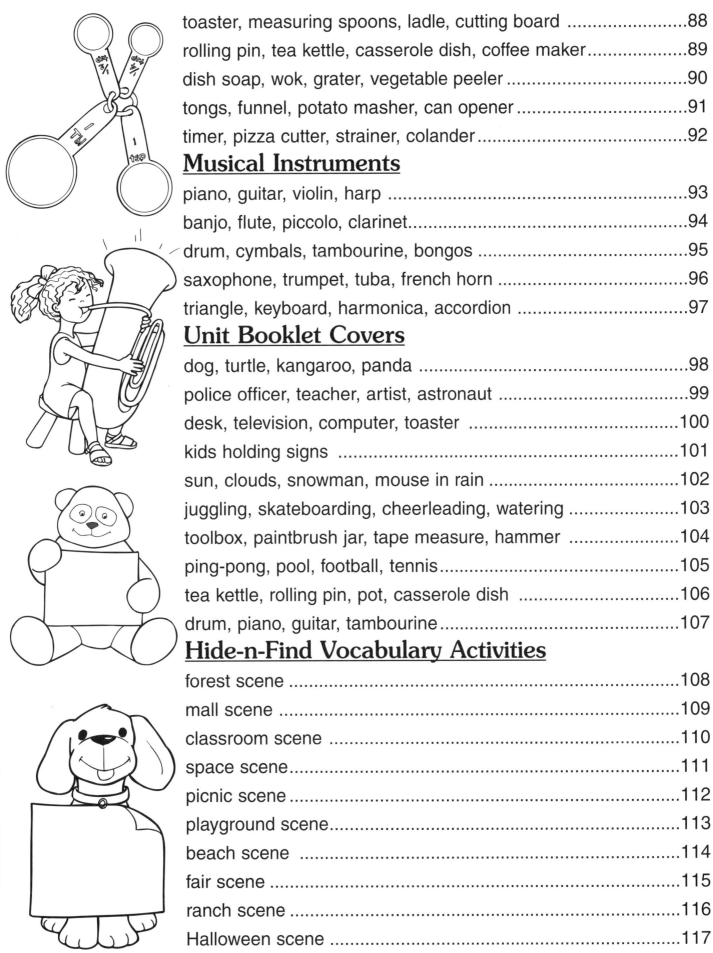

Musical Instruments

Unit Booklet Covers

Hide-n-Find Vocabulary Activities

©1997 Super Duper® Publications 1-800-277-8737

II. Concept Section

©1997 Super Duper® Publications 1-800-277-8737

III. Resource Section

©1997 Super Duper® Publications 1-800-277-8737

• • • • • • • Introduction • • • • • • •

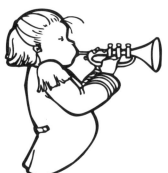

Basic Concept and Vocabulary Roundup is designed to help the busy Speech-Language Pathologist, Special Education Teacher and Bilingual/ ESL Specialist implement vocabulary and concept development components into their language program. This book contains 324 target vocabulary pictures, 224 target concept pictures, language bombardment sheets, hide-n-find picture activities, vocabulary analysis chart, sample lesson plan and parent letter, therapy ideas, unit booklet covers, motivational charts, reinforcement badges, and a variety of certificates. This comprehensive workbook is designed to combine both a remediation and parent involvement component, making the generalization process effective as well as fun.

This workbook was developed by a public school Speech-Language Pathologist who works with language delayed students. It is the intent of the author to package a motivational language program that is fun yet addresses both vocabulary and concept development. The illustrations of the target vocabulary and target concept pictures, as well as the language bombardment sheets, are humorous and provide numerous opportunities to reinforce a particular vocabulary word or concept. This makes the language development process motivating for the student, specialist, and parent!

The vocabulary section of this book includes 10 categories of commonly used words. The specialist may choose any number of target vocabulary pictures to present to the student in the remediation process. Once these target vocabulary words have been taught, they may be assembled on a ring and taken home for further practice. When the student returns for the following session, new target vocabulary words can be presented. Additionally, these new target words can be taught and added to those previously practiced.

Knowing the importance of concept development, the author felt it necessary to include a section of concept pictures. This allows a specialist the flexibility of working on vocabulary words and/or concepts throughout the remediation process. The concept section of this book includes both language bombardment sheets and target concept pictures. The auditory bombardment technique, taken from the phonological approach, has been found useful in language acquisition. (Further information on this

©1997 Super Duper® Publications 1-800-277-8737

phonological technique can be found in <u>Bombardment Bonanza</u>.) Reproducible language bombardment sentence sheets are provided to allow the specialist and parents the opportunity to model a particular concept for the child. These sheets have humorous illustrations surrounding the language bombardment sentences. They provide additional opportunities to reinforce a particular concept. The student can be encouraged to color the surrounding pictures at home. This makes the "read and listen" process a fun one!

The target concept pictures are designed to elicit a particular concept sentence structure from the child. Initially, the specialist chooses the appropriate target concept pictures for remediation use. The specialist then cuts out those particular pictures to be used in the language lesson. Once the pictures are produced, the specialist may choose to have the students color the target sentence pictures as a way of making the total experience more meaningful. The students then put their personalized colored pictures on a binder ring after subsequent lessons.

The target concept pictures along with the language bombardment sheets are to be sent home with the students. The parents/guardians can use these pictures and sheets to reinforce the language lesson. After the home follow-up activity, the students are asked to return the binder ring with the target concept pictures for future additions.

The <u>resource section</u> includes therapy ideas, reinforcement badges, motivational charts and certificates. These supplemental materials add fun to the learning of language!

<u>Basic Concept and Vocabulary Roundup</u> makes remediation more enjoyable for the specialist, student, and parent! Feel free to reproduce the worksheets as often as needed for classroom use.

Please remember that duplication for an entire school district or workshop is not permitted.

Bev

©1997 Super Duper® Publications 1-800-277-8737

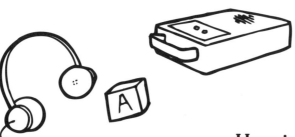
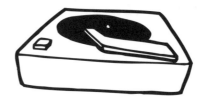
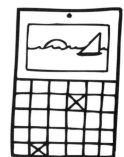

Here is a list of suggested materials we found helpful to begin our language program.

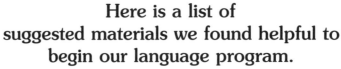

1. Headsets and microphone
2. Tape recorder
3. Record player
4. Classroom calendar to mark birthdays and holidays
5. Pocket chart for vocabulary words
6. Carpet squares for students to sit on
7. Storage bins for toys, manipulatives, puppets, etc.
8. Cubbies
9. Art supplies which could include: glue/glue sticks, glitter, yarn, cotton balls, construction paper, scissors, pencils, erasers, crayons, rulers, paint, paintbrushes, smocks, easels, stapler, felt pens, egg cartons, tongue depressors, paper plates, socks, pipe cleaners, ribbon, old material, etc.
10. Binder rings for vocabulary words
11. Assorted toys which could include: puppets, blocks, balls, puzzles, play dough, dolls, assorted stringing beads, stacking toys, cars, trucks, planes, etc.
12. Bean bags and bean bag board
13. Articles of clothing and costumes for make-believe play
14. Dollhouse and furniture
15. Plastic or wood stove set, plastic food and dishes
16. Variety of tables to include horse-shoe shaped table, round table for headsets, and a long rectangular table for art activities
17. Play phone
18. Records and cassette tapes of children's stories and songs
19. "Feely box"
20. Flannel board and flannel board stories
21. Instant Image camera and film
22. Mirrors
23. Book display case
24. Exercise mat
25. Outdoor equipment: tricycles, wagons, scooter, bicycles for older students, sandbox, rubber balls, hula hoops, sandbox toys
26. Old magazines and newspapers
27. Student chairs, children's beanbag chairs, and pillows
28. Face paints
29. Playhouse
30. Clothesline and clothespins to hang up wet paintings
31. Toy cash register, play money, and empty products containers
32. If possible, a classroom pet, (e.g., fish, hamster, hermit crabs, mouse, etc.)
33. Musical instruments
34. Rubber stamps and washable stamp pads

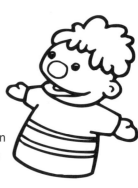
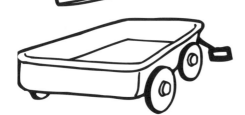
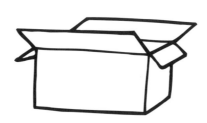
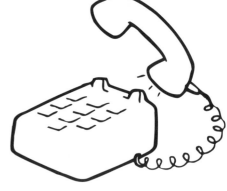

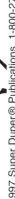

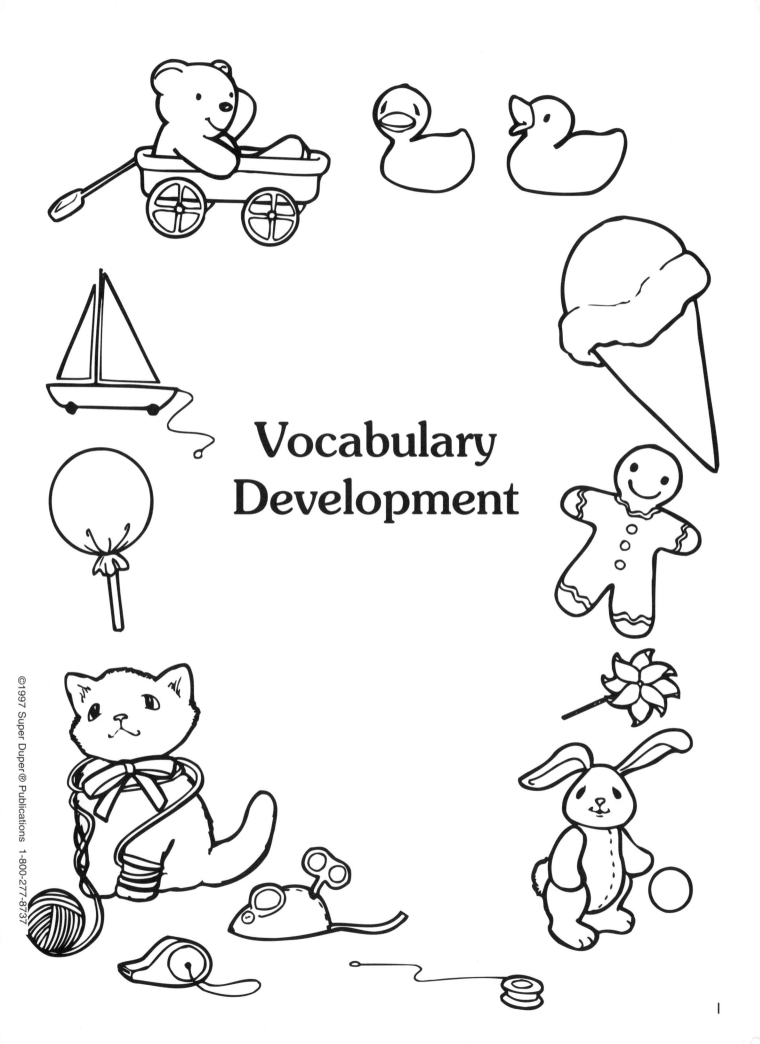

Vocabulary Development

How To Use The Vocabulary Section

Materials Needed:

- Paper cutter/scissors
- Duplicating paper (construction paper weight suggested)
- Hole punch
- Crayons or colored markers
- Optional: laminating paper/film
- Binder rings

Directions:

1. After duplicating selected target words, cut the pictures apart using the dotted lines as a guide. The child can color target pictures.

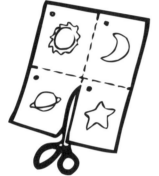

2. Hole punch each picture in the upper left hand corner through the printed circle.

3. Have child select a front cover design. Child can use crayons or markers to decorate it. Laminate for durability.

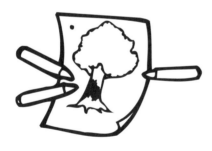

4. Repeat hole punch procedure (see step #2) for child's front cover.

5. Attach front cover and target words to a 1" to 2 1/2" ring. Ring size will depend on the number of target words.

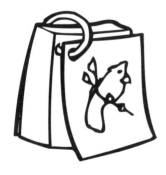

6. Continue to add pages after each therapy session.

*Note: The motivational charts on pages 240-241 can also be attached to the ring. Mini incentive stickers are perfect rewards for these charts.

©1997 Super Duper® Publications 1-800-277-8737

Analysis Chart of Students' Vocabulary Scores

Students' Names	Animals/ Pets		Body Parts		Furniture, Appliances & Accessories		Occupations		Weather Words		Verbs		Tools		Sports		Kitchen Items & Eating Utensils		Musical Instruments		Comments
	Pre	Post	Pre	Post	Pre	Post	Pre	Post	Pre	Post	Pre	Post	Pre	Post	Pre	Post	Pre	Post	Pre	Post	
Date																					
Date																					
Date																					
Date																					
Date																					
Date																					
Date																					
Date																					
Date																					
Date																					

Sample Lesson Plan
Unit: Animals/Pets
Words: Rat, Mouse, Lizard, Fish

Language Lesson

8:30-8:40   Students arrive to class

8:40-8:55   Circle time begins—Review previous session words and introduce new words

- Teach the nursery rhymes "Hickory, Dickory, Dock" and "Three Blind Mice"
- Have students march and sing to the "Mickey Mouse Parade" theme song
- Have students pretend to fish using a toy fishing pole with a magnet placed at the end. The students will catch different colored construction paper fish with paper clips attached. Once the fish is caught, the student will verbalize the color and the word fish, for example "blue fish."

8:55-9:10   Half of the students go to the "Listening Center" to put on their headphones and listen to the names of the four animals/pets. Then the story, One Fish, Two Fish, Red Fish, Blue Fish by Dr. Seuss is read by the teacher through the headsets.

- The other half of the students go to the art table to name and color their four target vocabulary pictures. When the coloring is completed, the teacher places the finished pictures on the students' rings to take home after the session.

9:10-9:20   A small aquarium with any of the above animals will be brought to school for the students to observe. (If possible, a pet shop employee could bring several animals to the class and talk to the students about them.) Students will draw a picture of the animal they see.

9:20-9:30   Snack (fish crackers and juice) and then Bathroom Break

9:30-9:45   Outside or inside play

9:45-10:00 Students will ask for an animal stamp (i.e. mouse or lizard) and then get to stamp it on a piece of paper.

- Students will sponge paint using a "rat" or a "fish" shaped sponge dipped into paint and then pressed onto construction paper or tag board.

10:00-10:15 Students will listen to the story, If You Give A Mouse A Cookie by Laura Joffe Numeroff.

4

- Using four milk bottles with the target vocabulary words attached, the students will try to drop clothespins in the milk bottles. If the student gets a clothespin in, she/he will name the picture.

10:15-10:25 Students will throw beanbags on one of the four target vocabulary pictures and then name which animal/pet the beanbag lands on.

- Students return to the "Listening Center" to review the four target vocabulary words.

- Students phone on a pretend telephone to their best friend or relatives and name their four target vocabulary words.

10:25-10:30 Students pack up and go home.

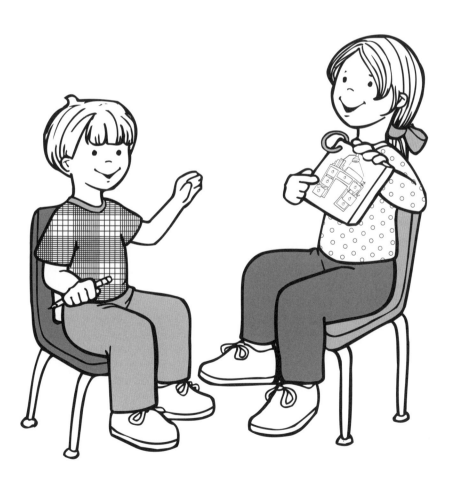

School District/Private Clinic
Home Speech Program

Date: _____
Unit: Animals/Pets
Vocabulary Words: Mouse, Rat, Fish, Lizard

Dear Parents,

Today in class your child participated in the following activities:

1. We learned two nursery rhymes—"Hickory, Dickory, Dock" and "Three Blind Mice."
2. We listened to two stories: <u>One Fish, Two Fish, Red Fish, Blue Fish</u> by Dr. Seuss and <u>If You Give A Mouse A Cookie</u> by Laura Joffe Numeroff.
3. We watched a lizard (or a fish) in an aquarium and drew a picture of the animal.
4. We sponge painted using sponges in the shape of fish or rats.

• For homework, please ask your child to name the vocabulary words on his/her ring. Ask your child which animal/pet is his/her favorite and why.

Additional Suggestions:
1. Visit a pet store and have your child name as many pets as they can.
2. Visit a local library and pick out a book on one of the animals we talked about today in class.
3. Visit an aquarium and discuss the different types and colors of fish.

©1997 Super Duper® Publications 1-800-277-8737

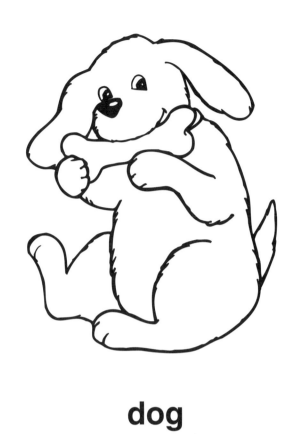

dog

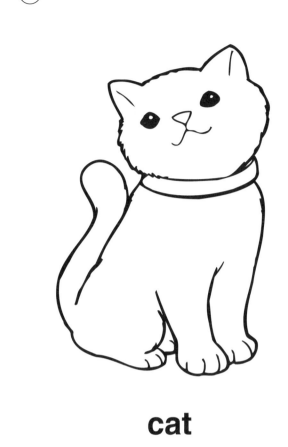

cat

© 1997 Super Duper® Publications 1-800-277-8737

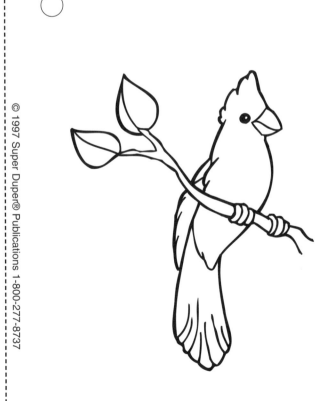

bird

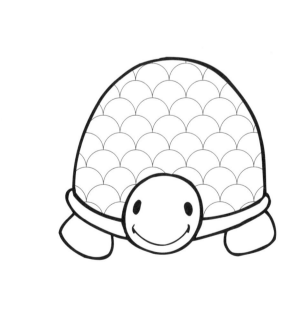

turtle

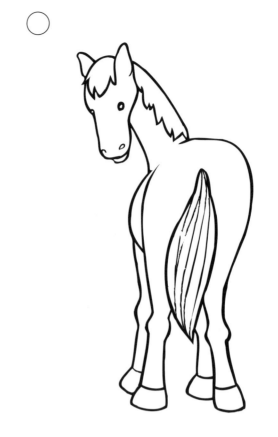
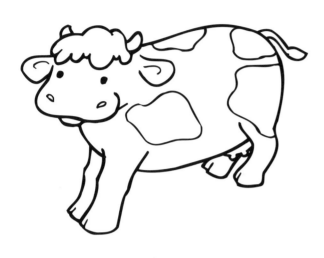

cow

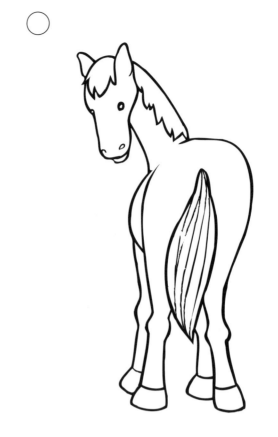

horse

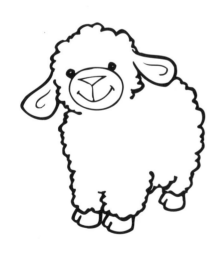

sheep

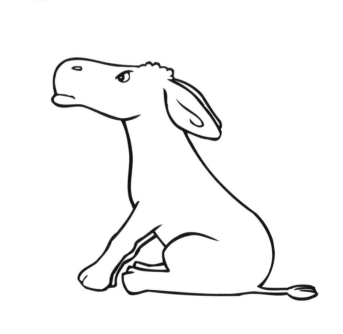

donkey

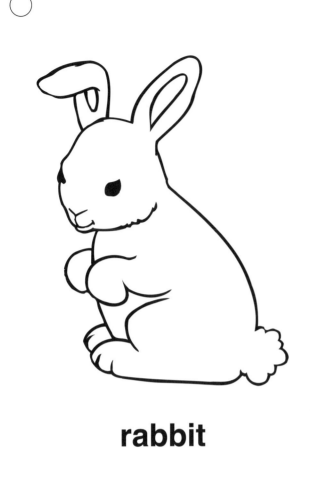

rabbit

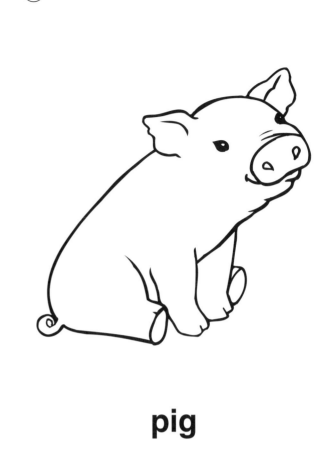

pig

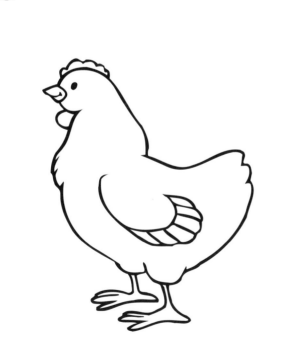

chicken

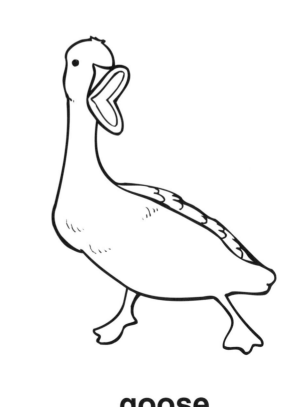

goose

9

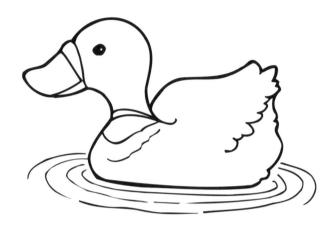

duck

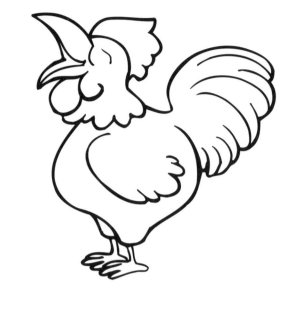

rooster

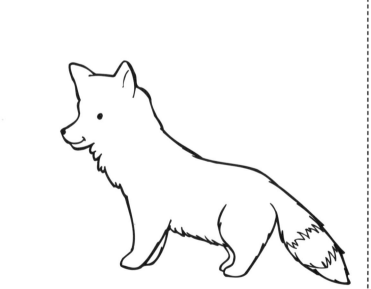

fox

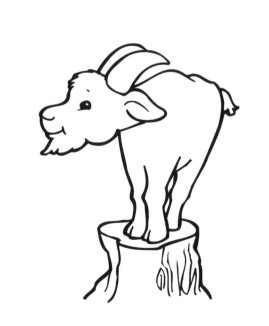

goat

© 1997 Super Duper® Publications 1-800-277-8737

rat

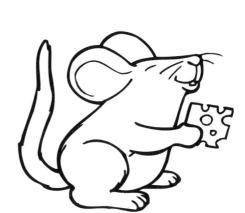

mouse

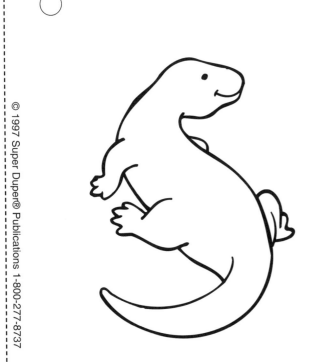

lizard

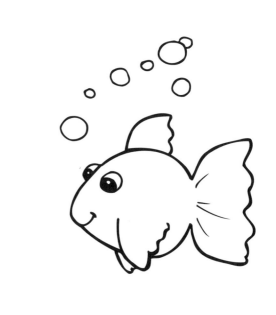

fish

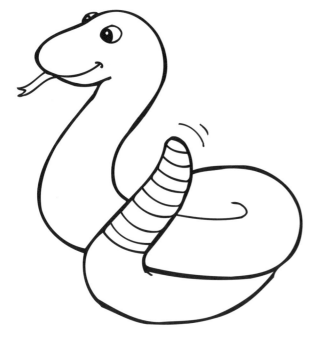

snake

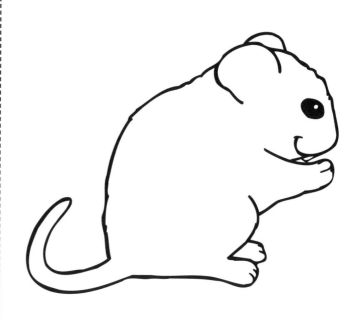

hamster

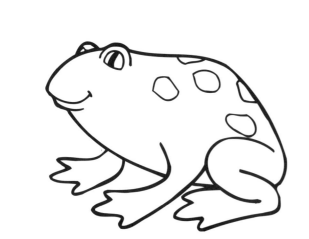

frog

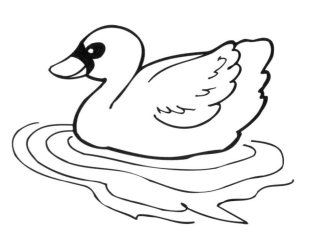

swan

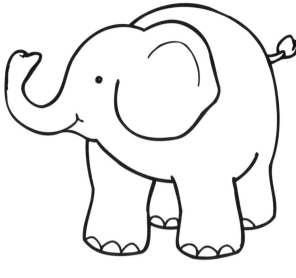

elephant

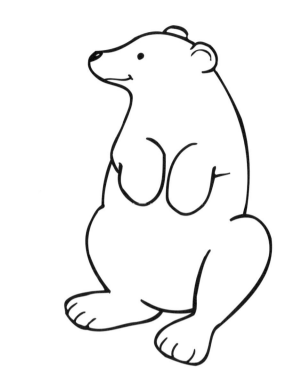

bear

© 1997 Super Duper® Publications 1-800-277-8737

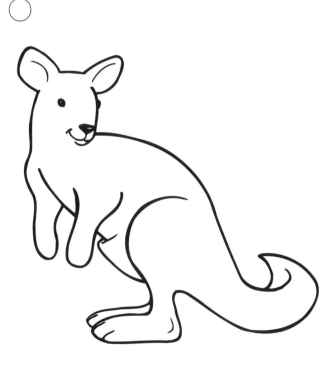

kangaroo

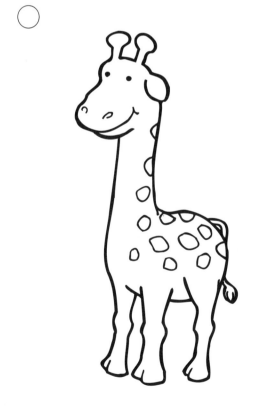

giraffe

13

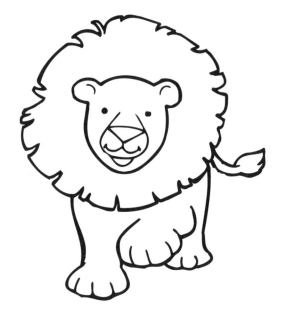

lion

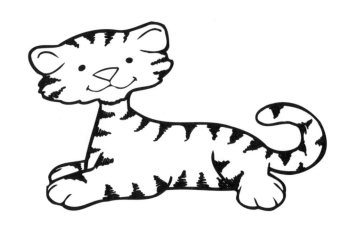

tiger

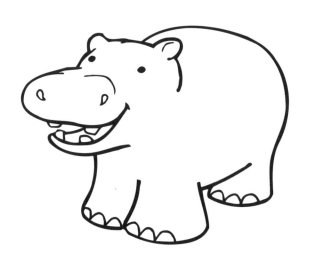

hippopotamus

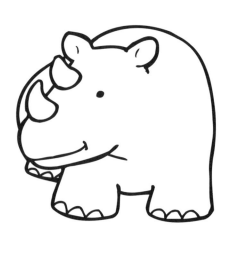

rhinoceros

14

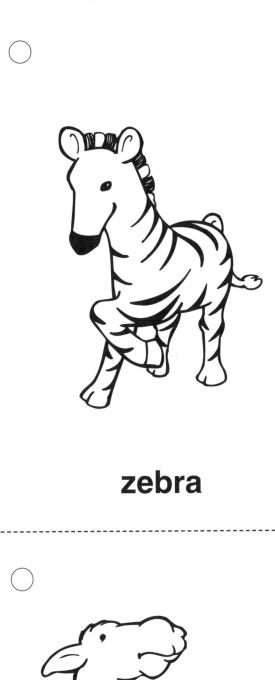

zebra

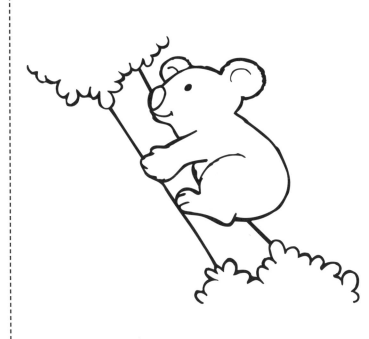

koala

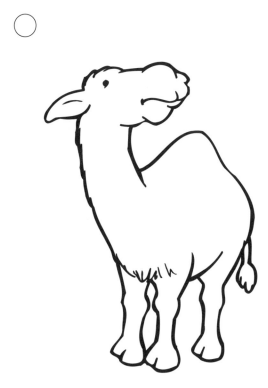

camel

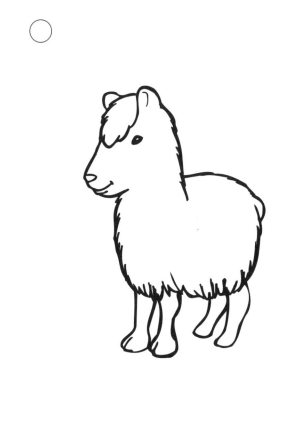

llama

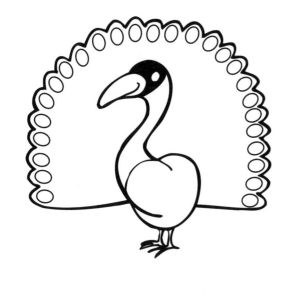

peacock

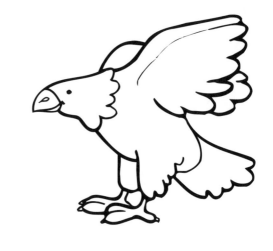

eagle

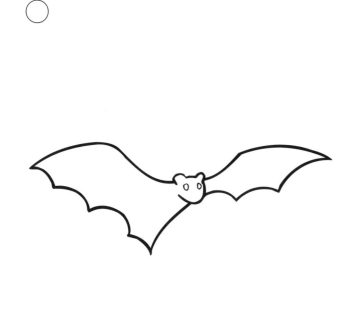

bat

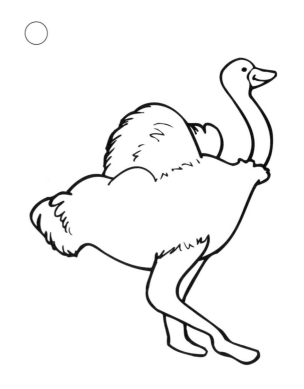

ostrich

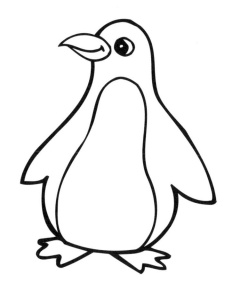

penguin

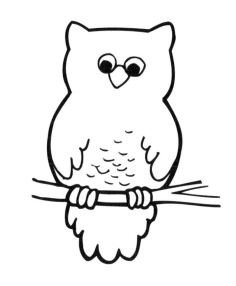

owl

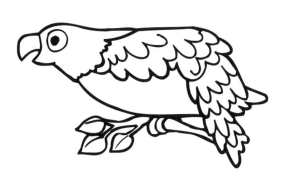

parrot

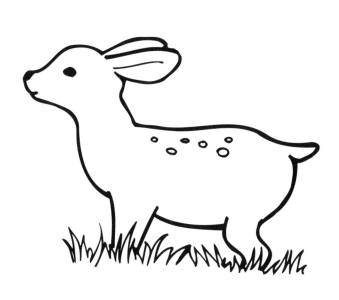

deer

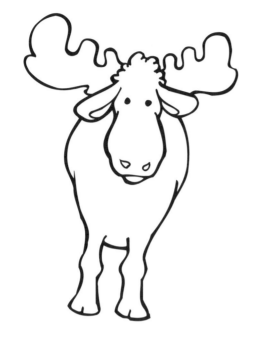

moose

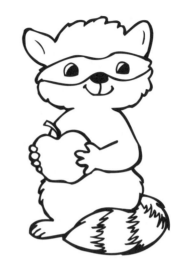

raccoon

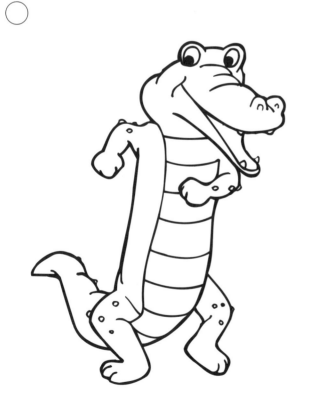

alligator

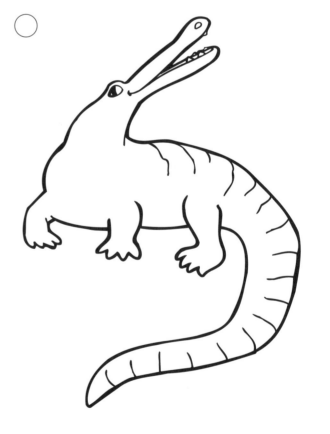

crocodile

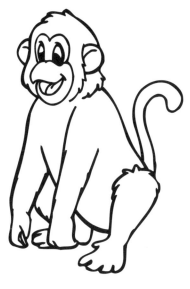

monkey

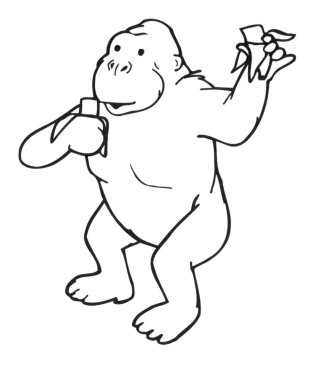

gorilla

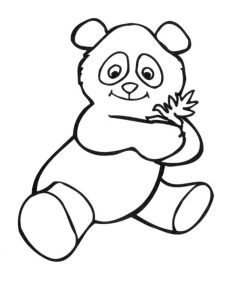

panda bear

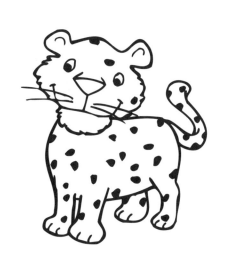

leopard

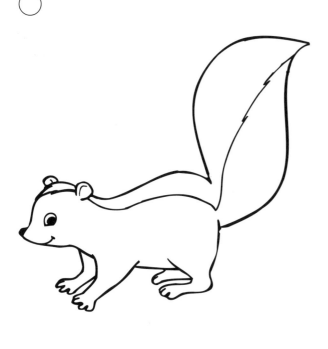

skunk

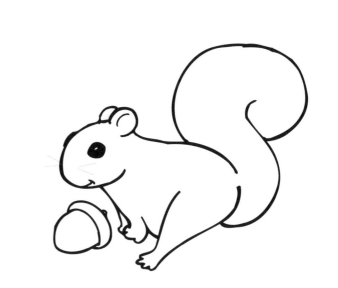

squirrel

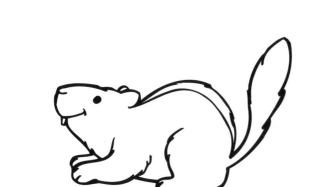

chipmunk

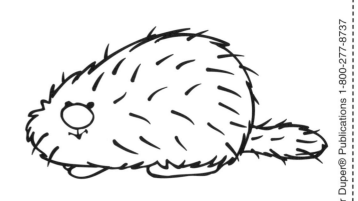

porcupine

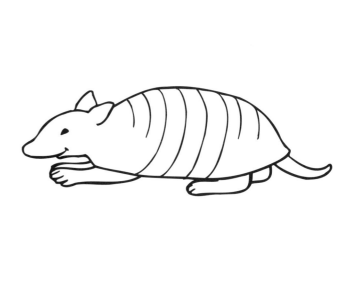

wolf

armadillo

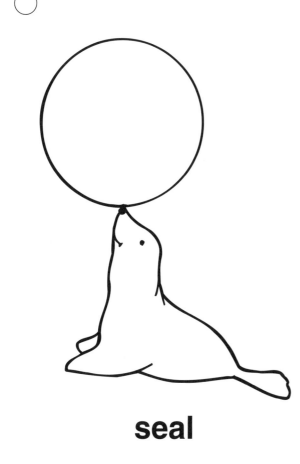

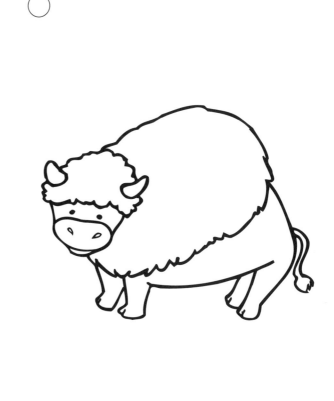

seal

bison

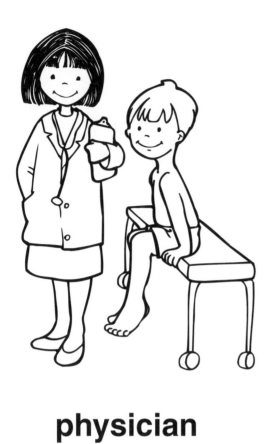

physician

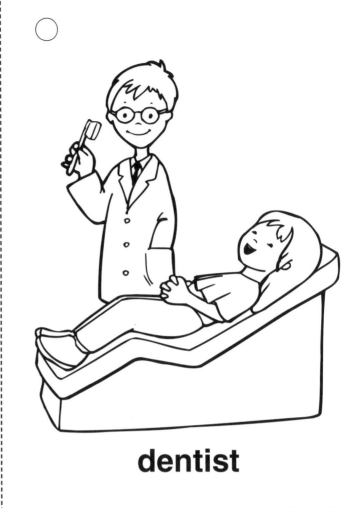

dentist

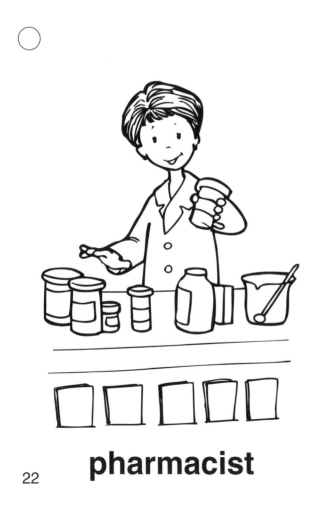

pharmacist

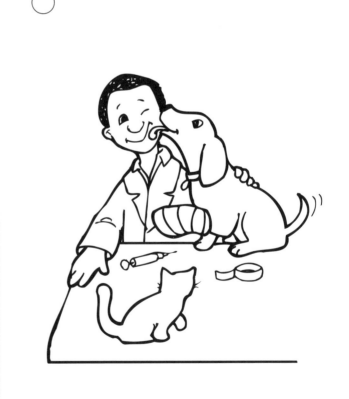

veterinarian

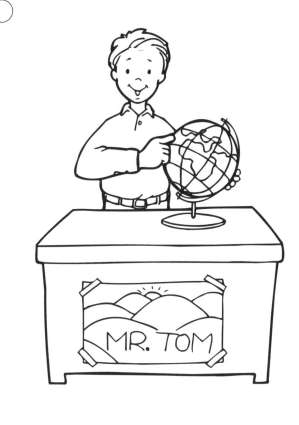

teacher

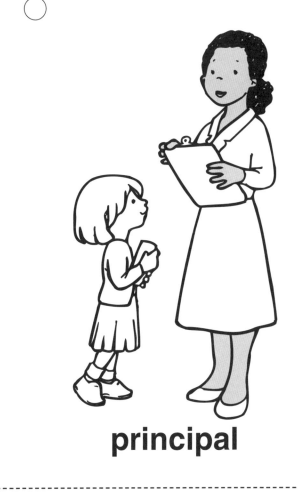

principal

© 1997 Super Duper® Publications 1-800-277-8737

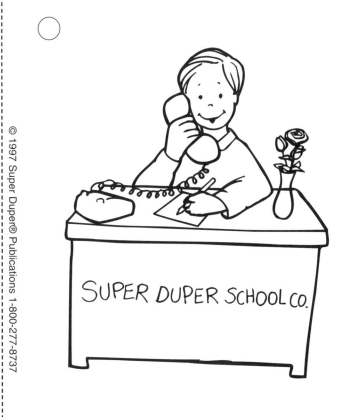

secretary

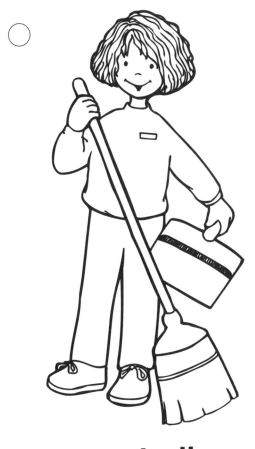

custodian

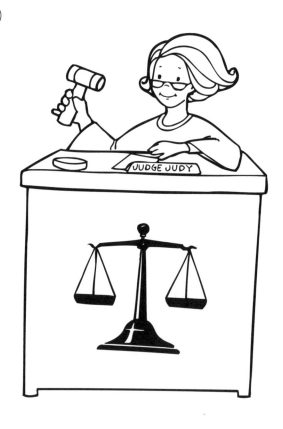

judge

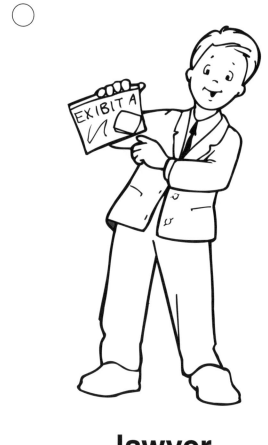

lawyer

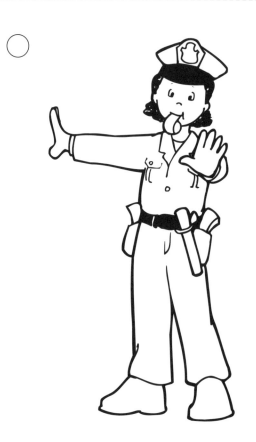

police officer

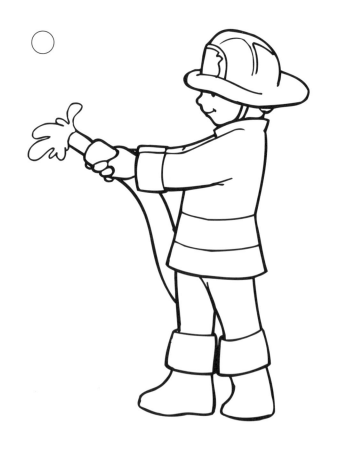

fire fighter

Cut pictures apart on dotted line

© 1997 Super Duper® Publications 1-800-277-8737

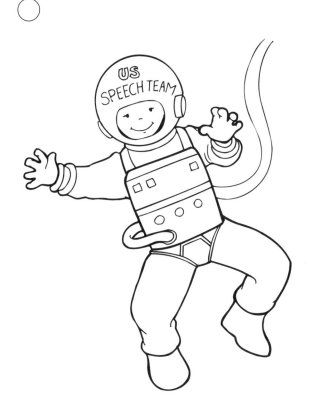

astronaut

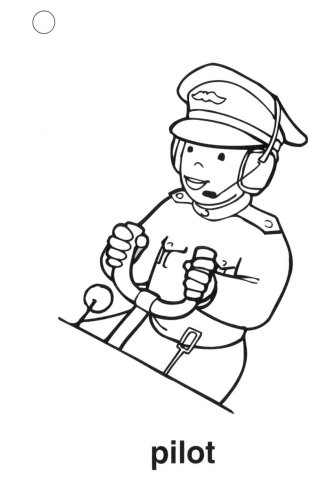

pilot

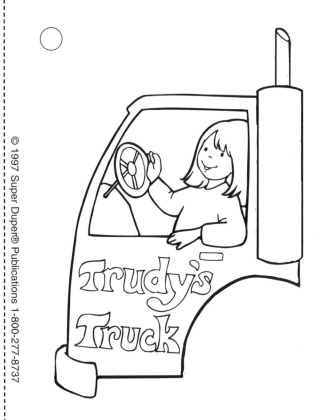

truck driver

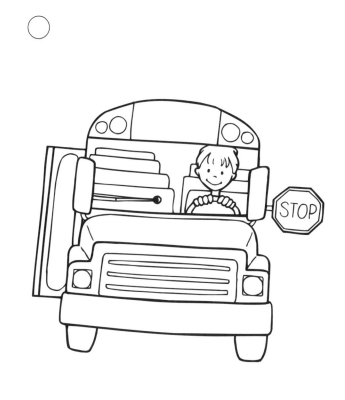

bus driver

25

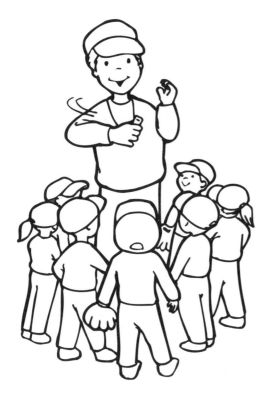

coach

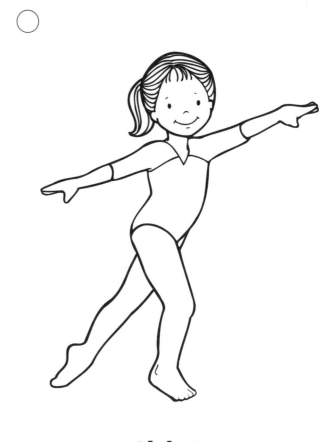

athlete

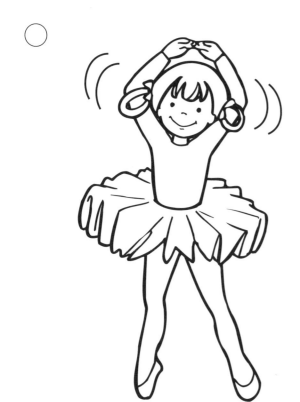

dancer

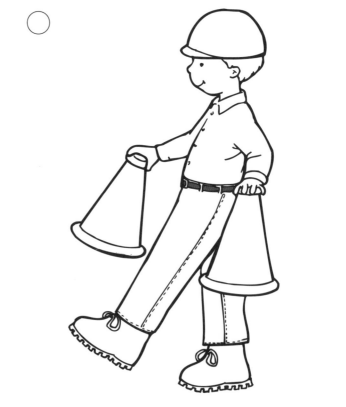

construction worker

© 1997 Super Duper® Publications 1-800-277-8737

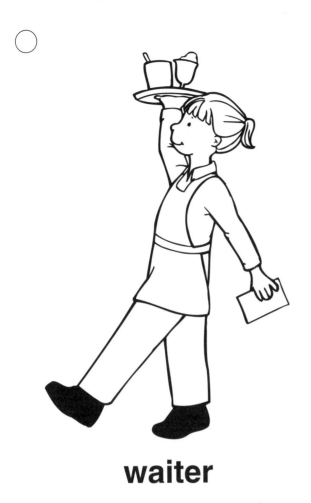

waiter

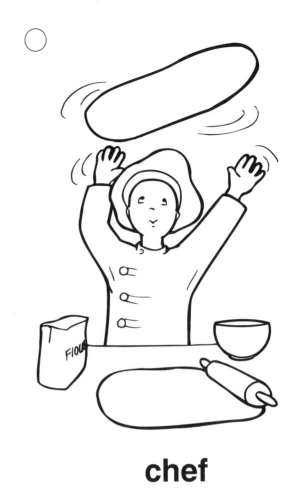

chef

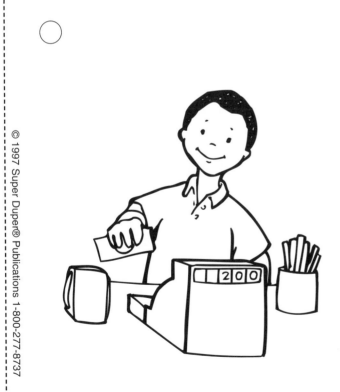

cashier

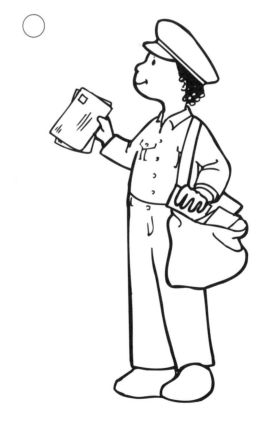

mail carrier

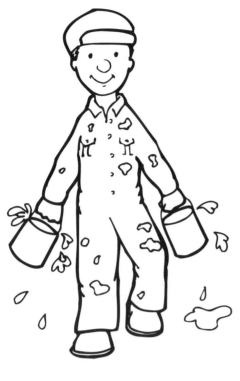

painter

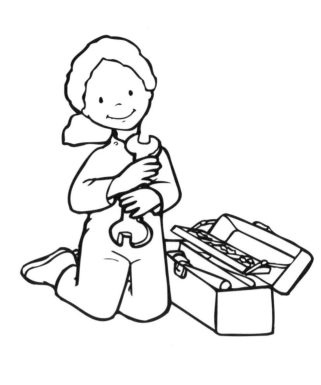

mechanic

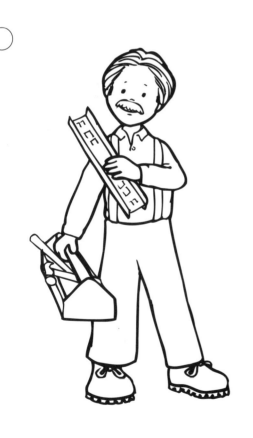

carpenter

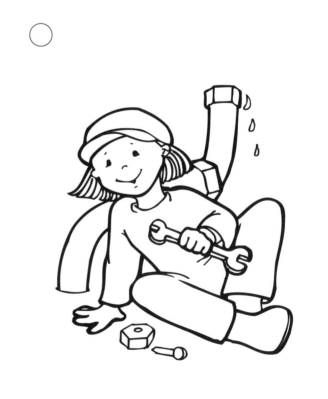

plumber

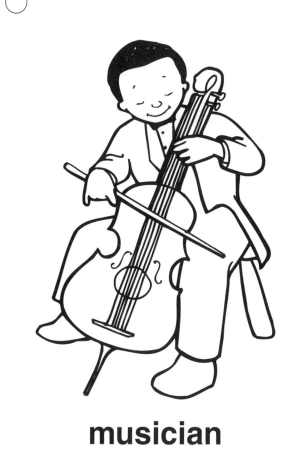

musician

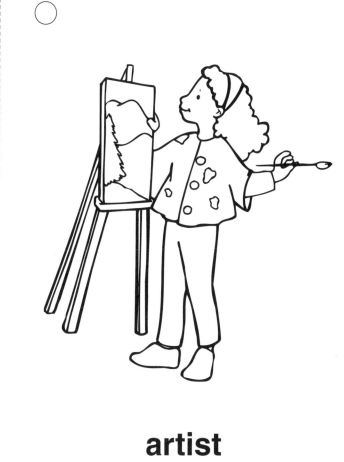

artist

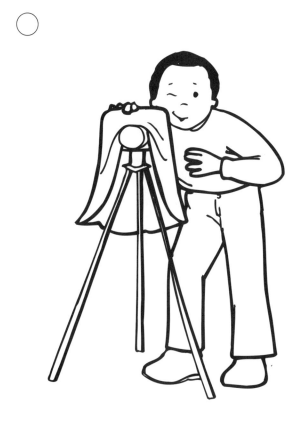

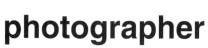

photographer

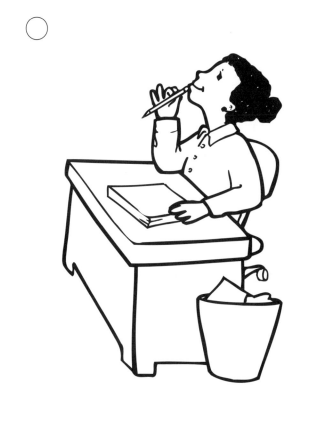

author

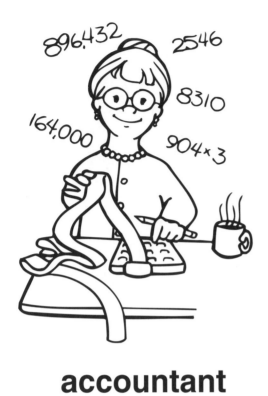

accountant

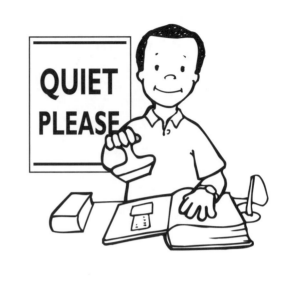

librarian

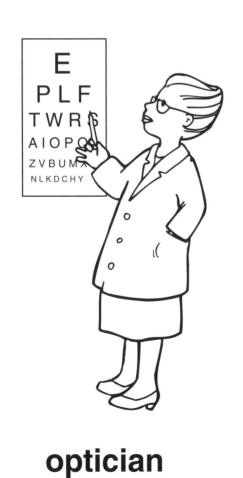

optician

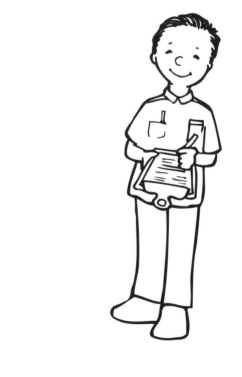

nurse

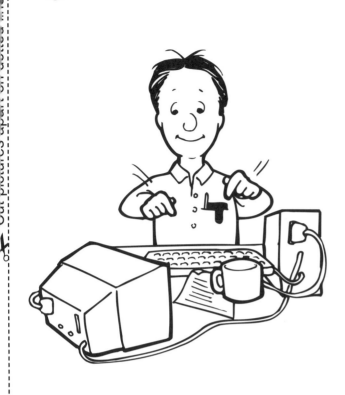

computer programmer

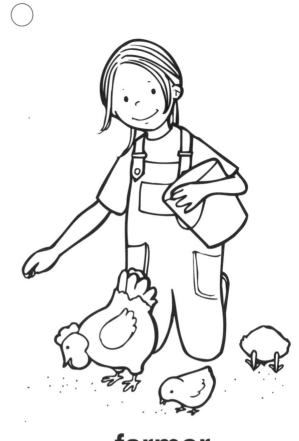

farmer

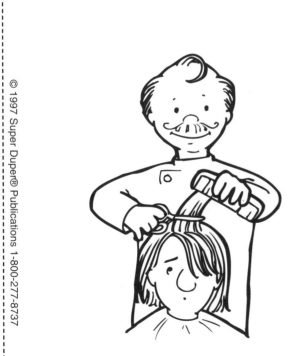

barber

hair stylist

31

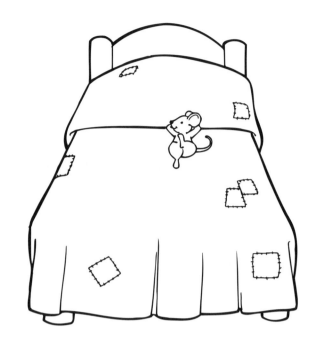

bed

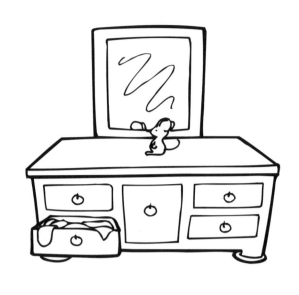

dresser

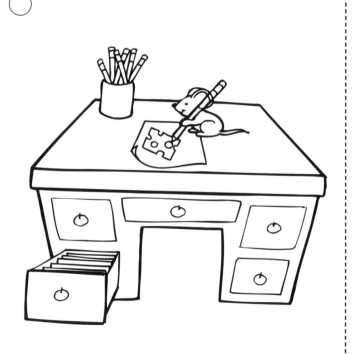

desk

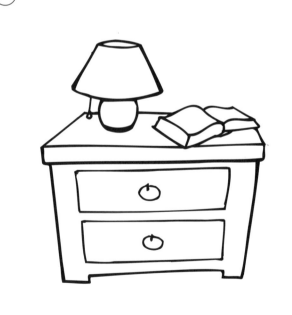

nightstand

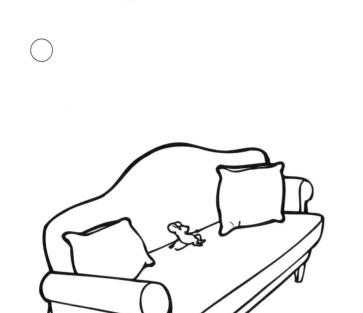

couch

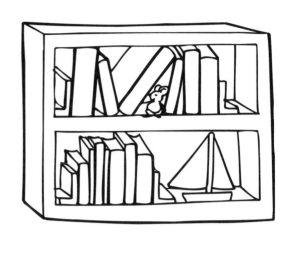

bookshelf

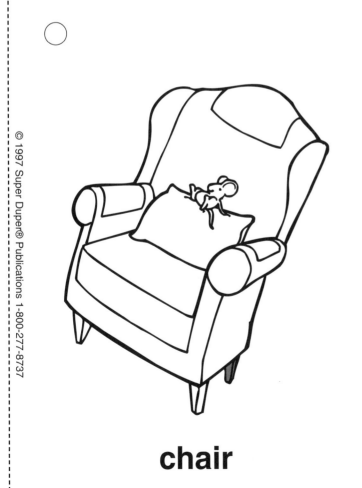

chair

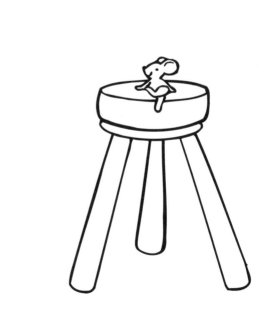

stool

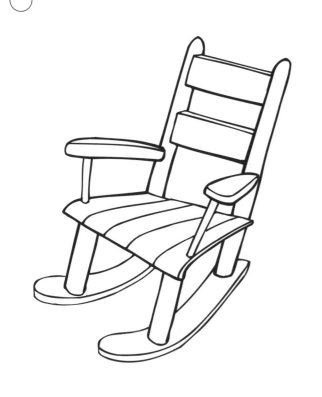

rocking chair

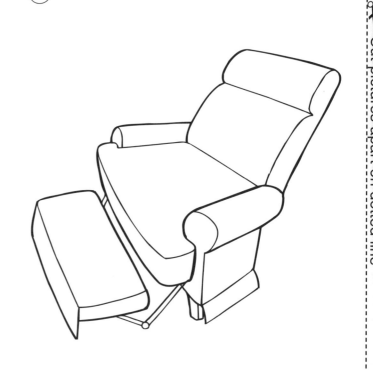

recliner

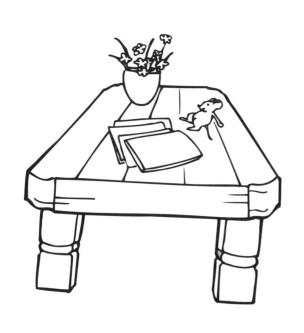

coffee table

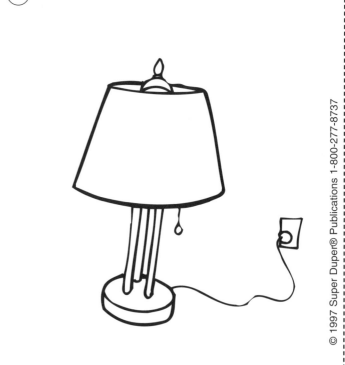

lamp

34

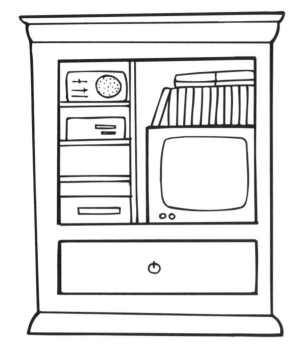

entertainment center

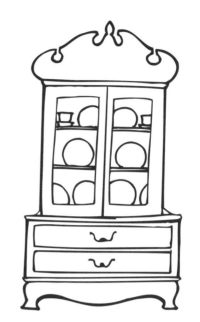

hutch

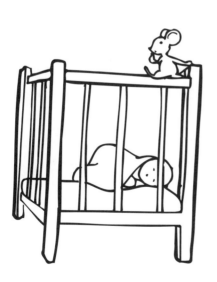

crib

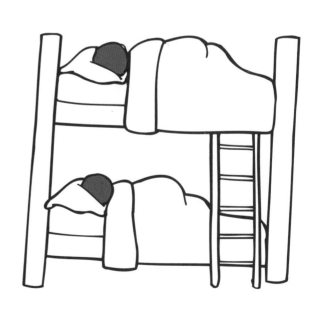

bunk beds

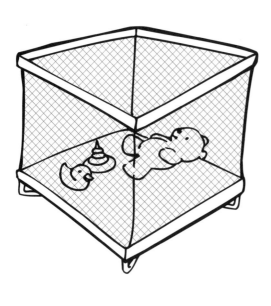

playpen

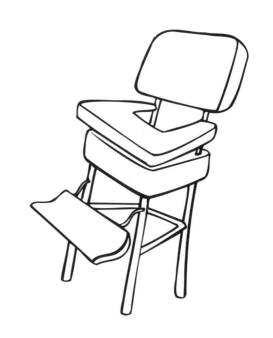

high chair

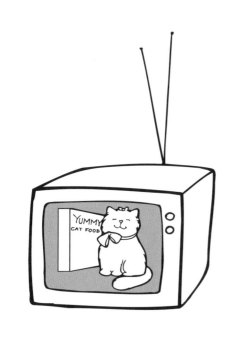

television

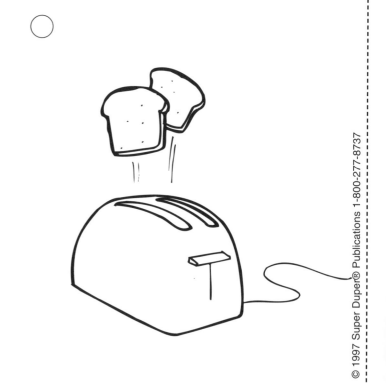

toaster

Cut pictures apart on dotted line

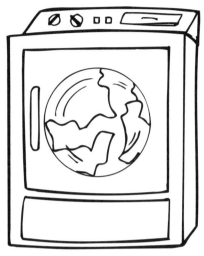

dryer

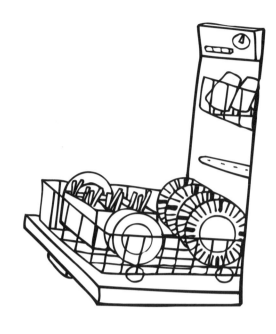

dishwasher

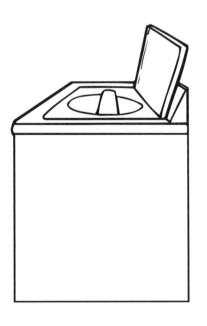

washer

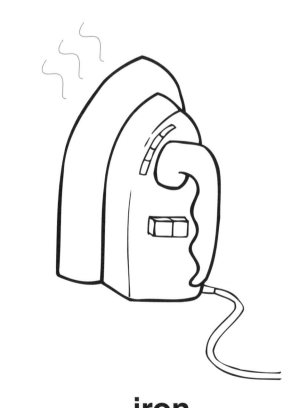

iron

DVD player

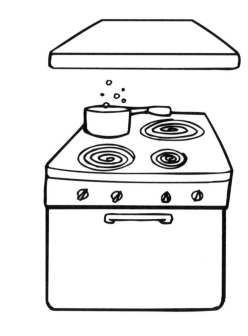

stove

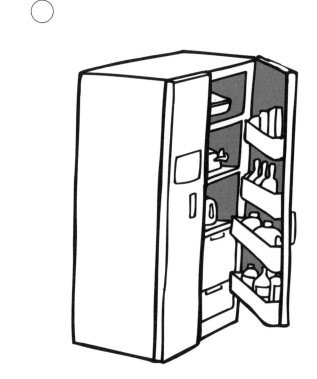

refrigerator

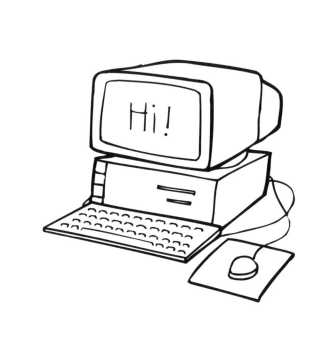

computer

© 1997 Super Duper® Publications 1-800-277-8737

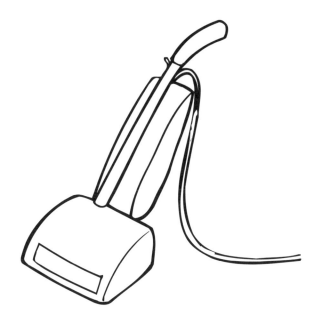

vacuum cleaner

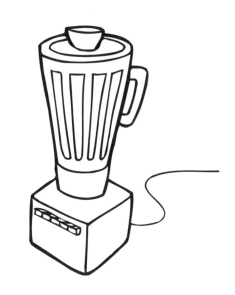

blender

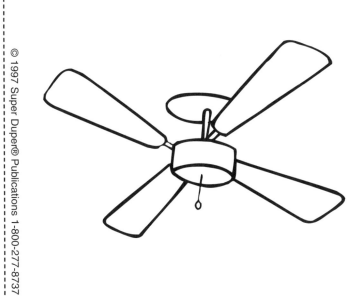

ceiling fan

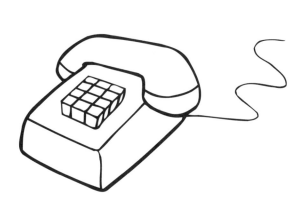

telephone

39

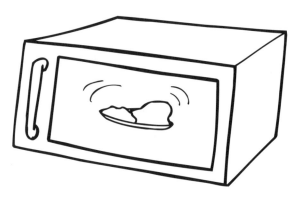

microwave oven

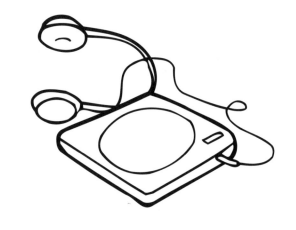

stereo/headset

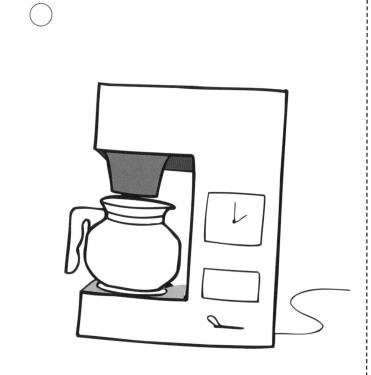

coffee maker

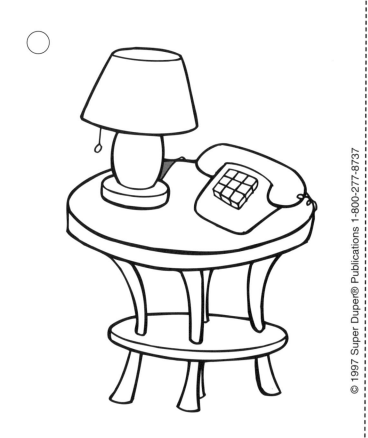

end table

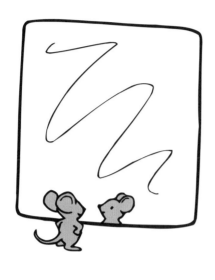

mirror

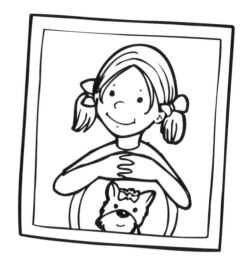

picture

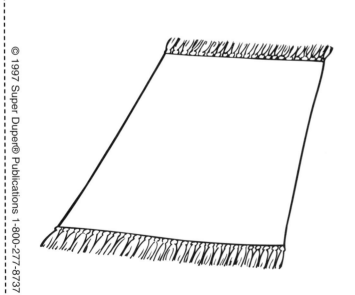

rug

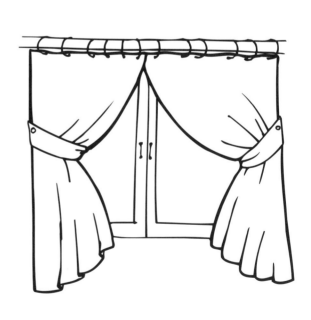

curtains

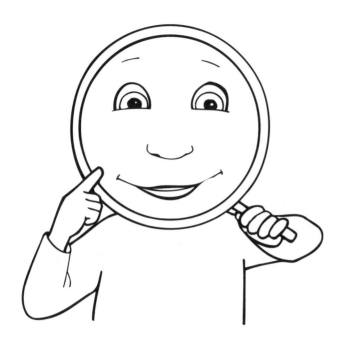

face

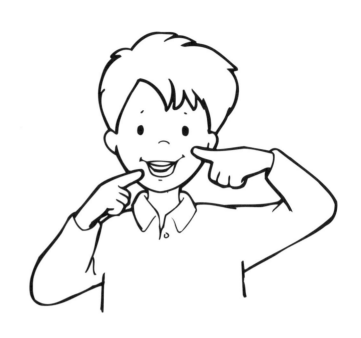

mouth

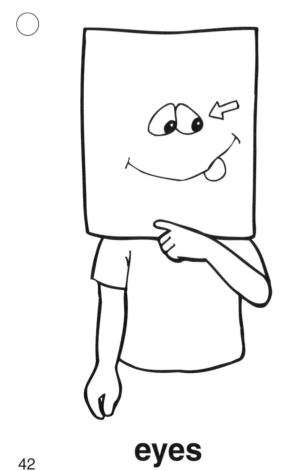

eyes

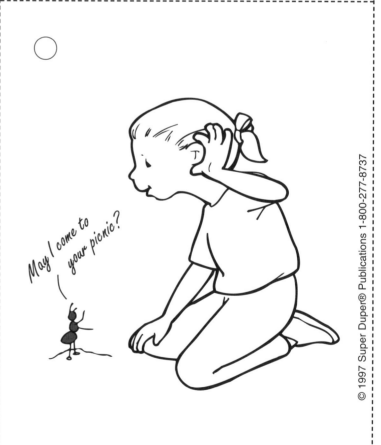

May I come to your picnic?

ear

42

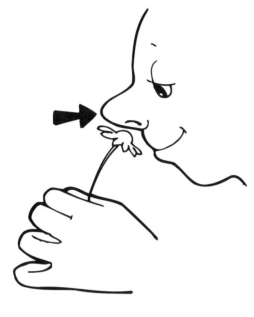

nose

eyebrow

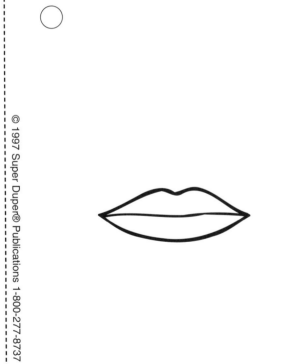

lips

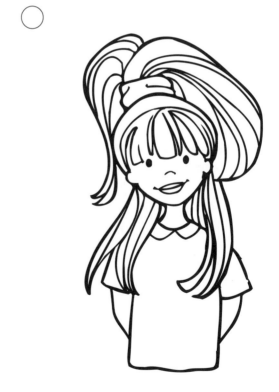

hair

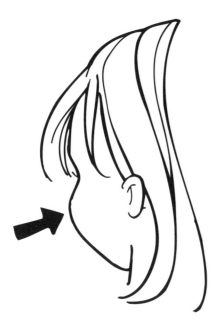

cheek

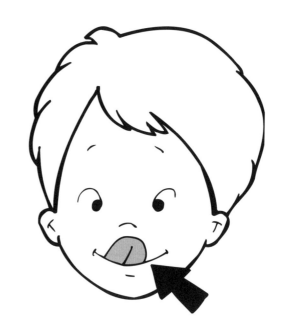

tongue

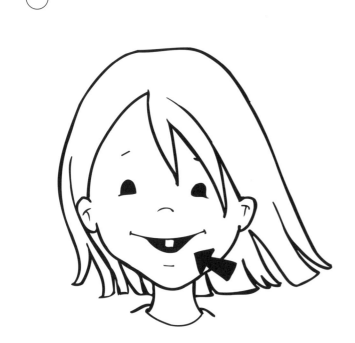

tooth

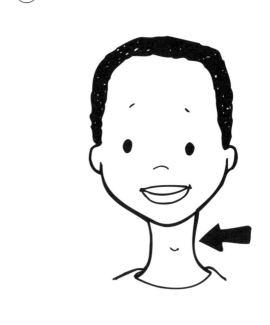

neck

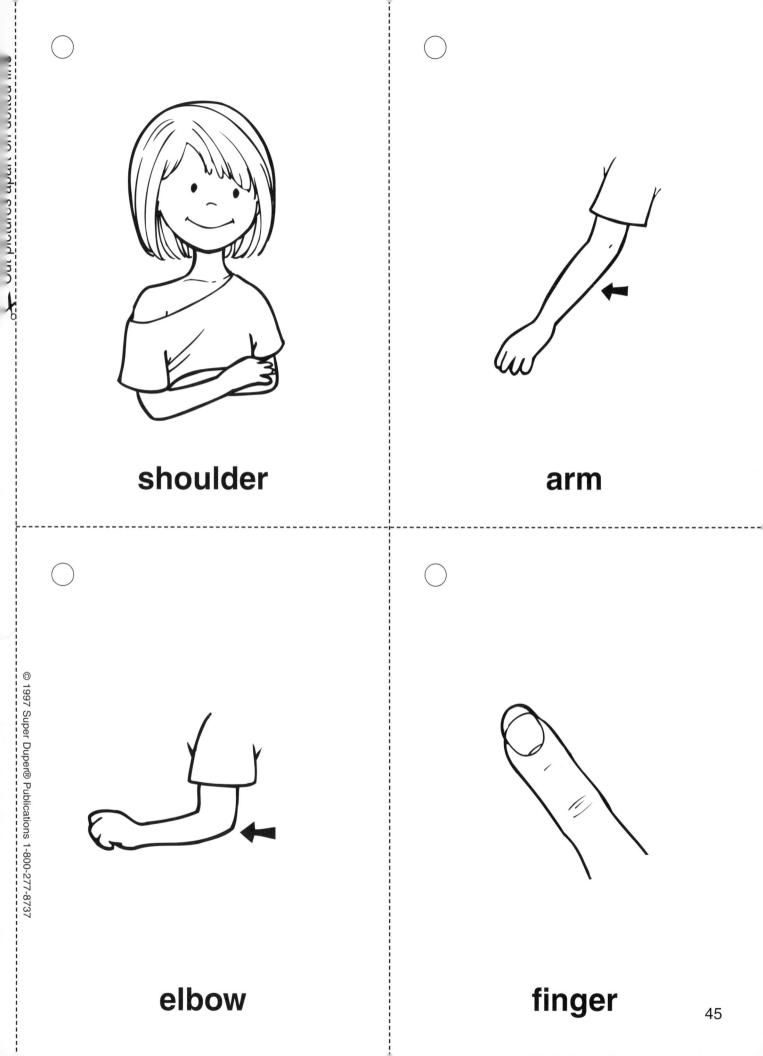

shoulder

arm

elbow

finger

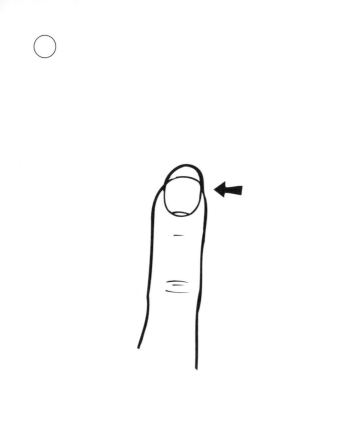

fingernail

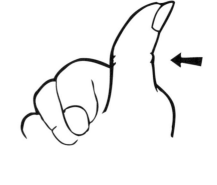

thumb

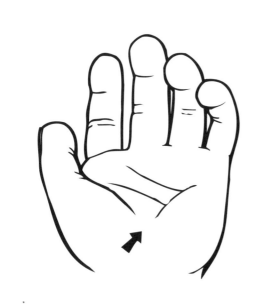

palm

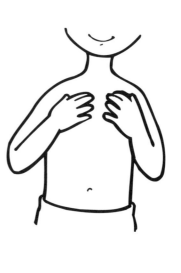

chest

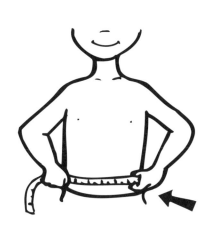

back

waist

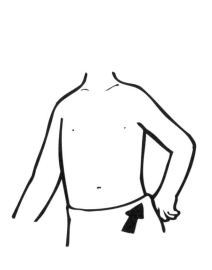

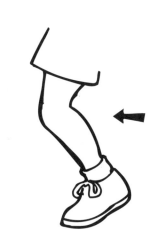

hip

leg

47

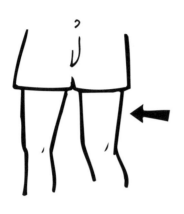

thigh

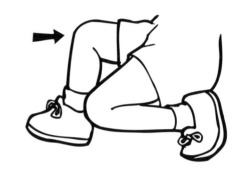

knee

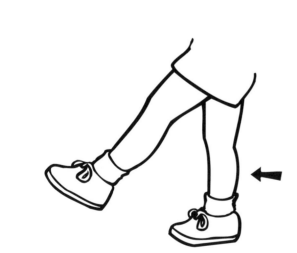

calf

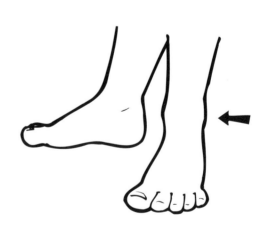

ankle

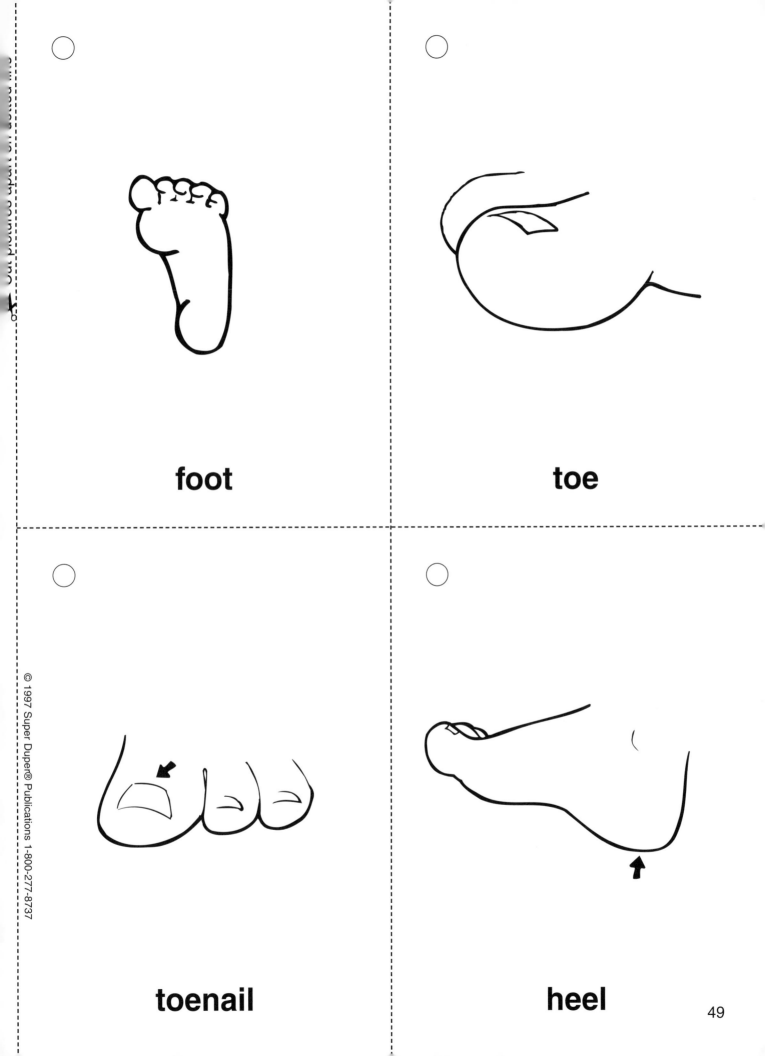

foot

toe

toenail

heel

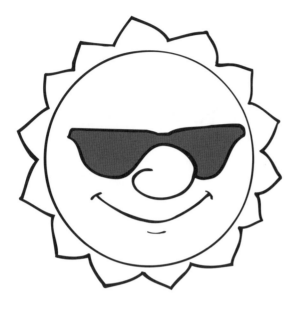

sun

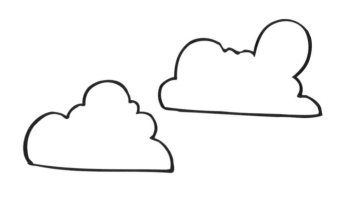

clouds

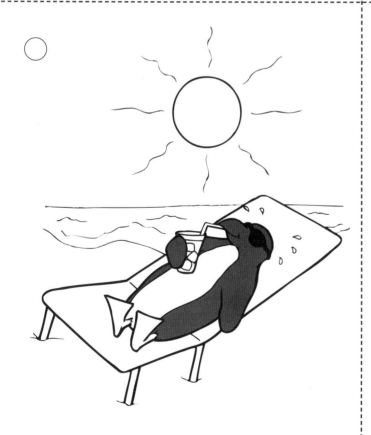

hot

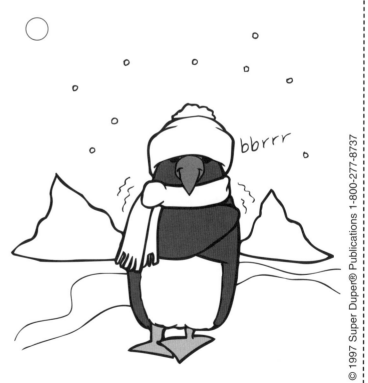

cold

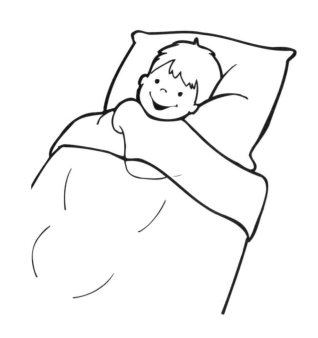

warm

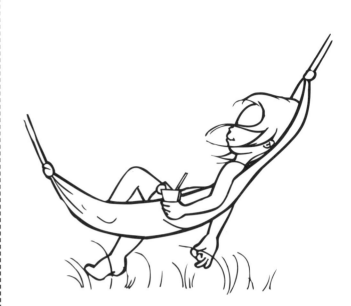

cool

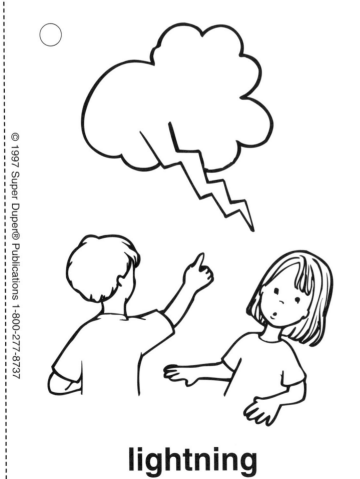

lightning

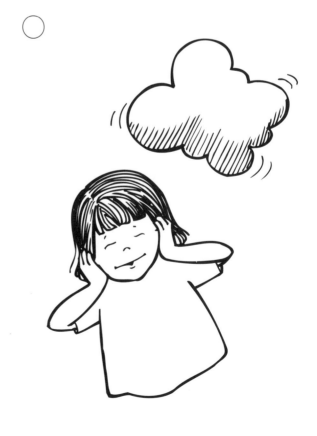

thunder

51

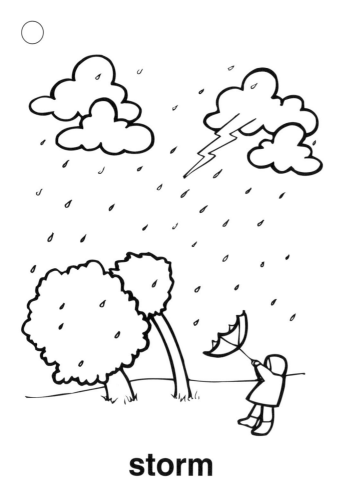

storm

rain

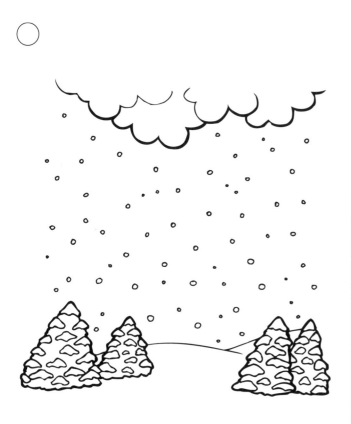

snow

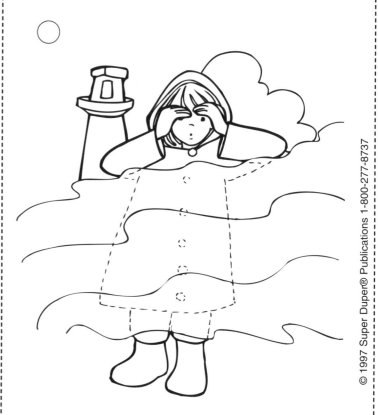

fog

52

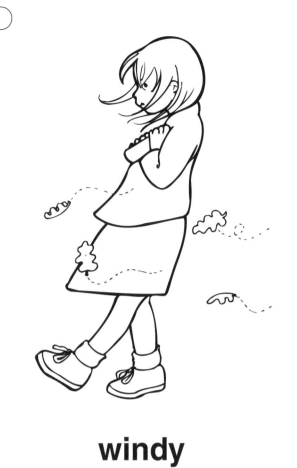

windy

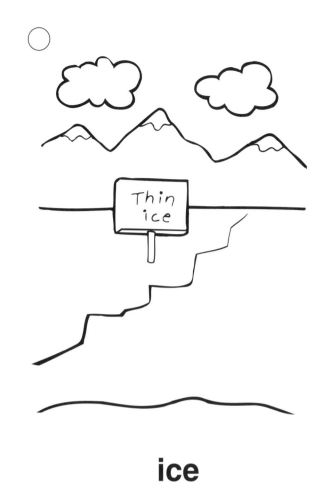

ice

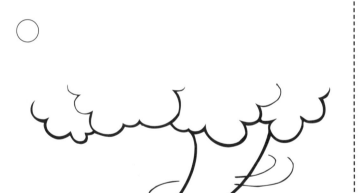

tornado

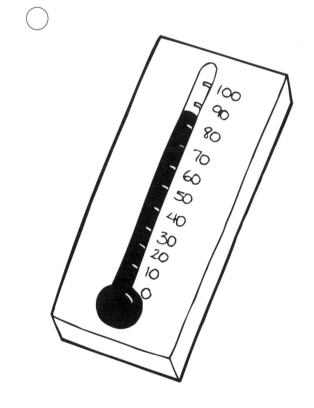

thermometer

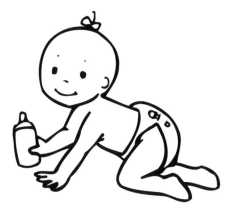

crawl

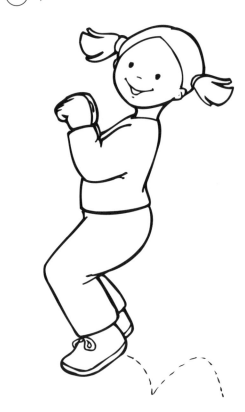

hop

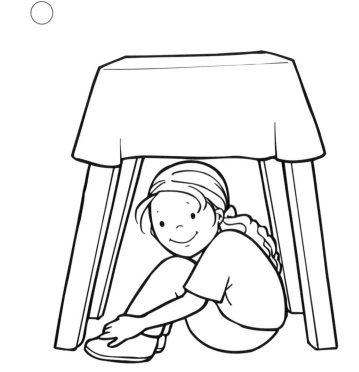

hide

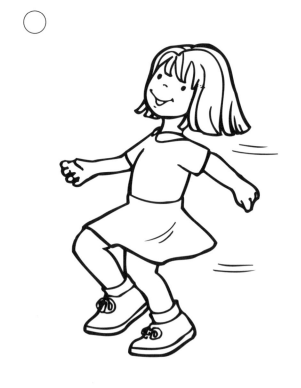

skip

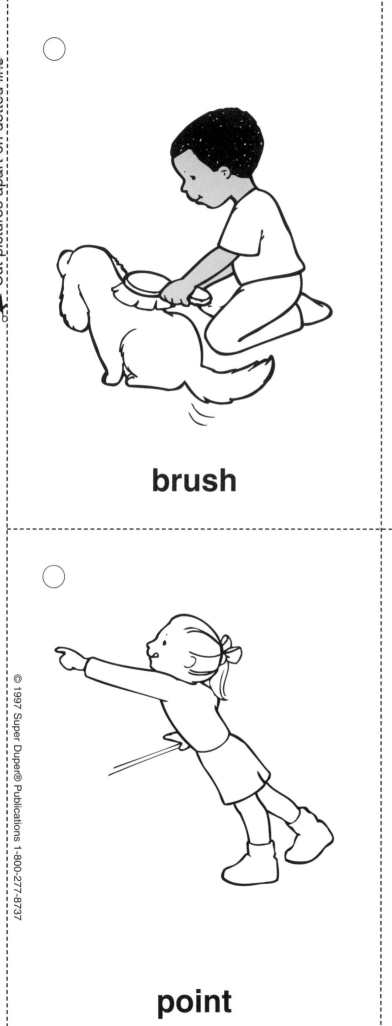

brush

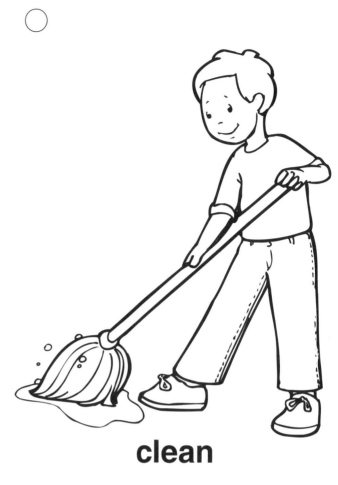

clean

point

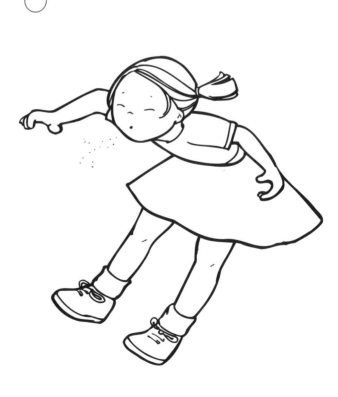

sneeze

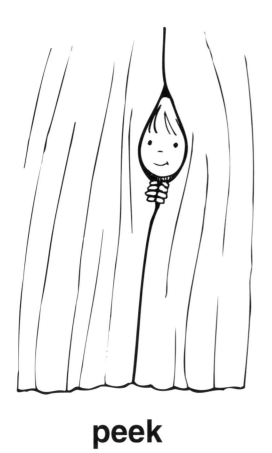

peek

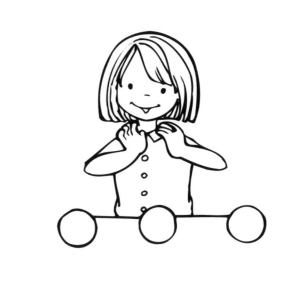

clap

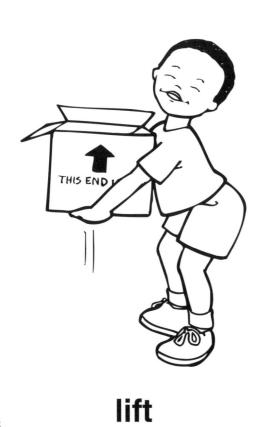

lift

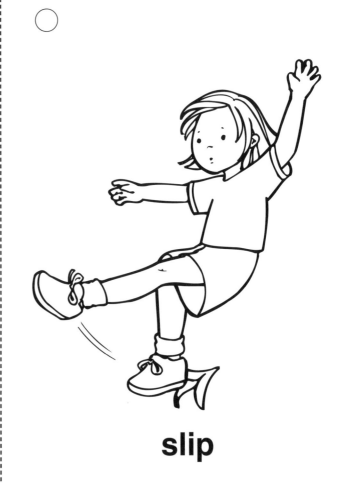

slip

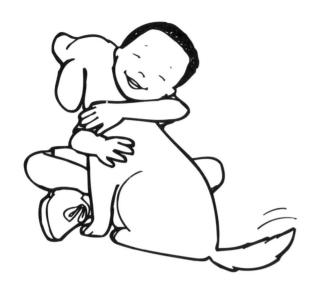

hug

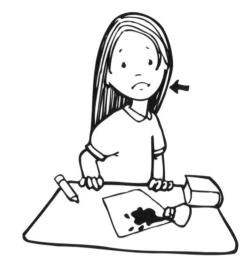

frown

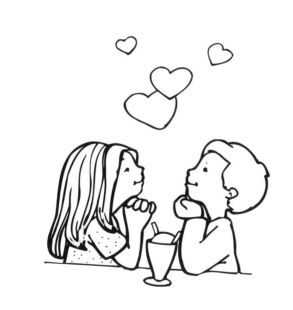

love

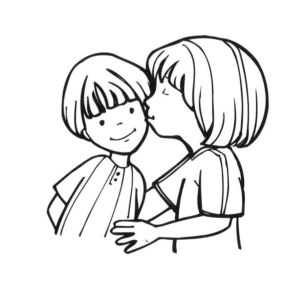

kiss

57

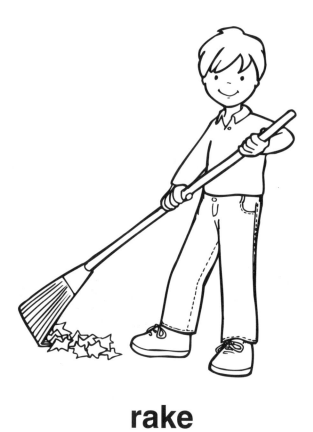

rake

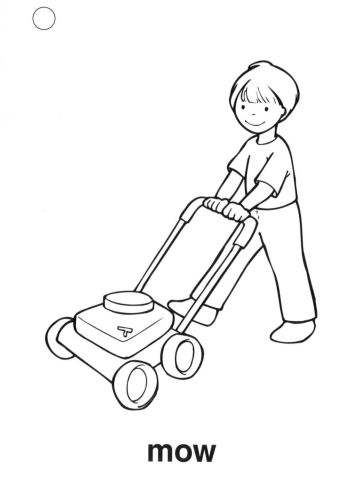

mow

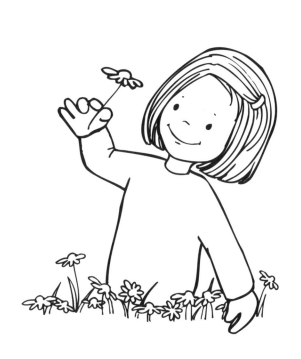

pick

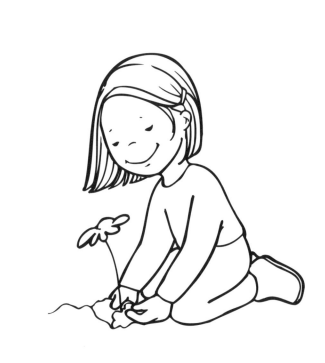

plant

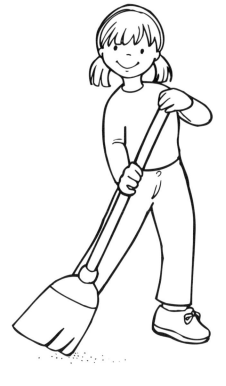

sweep

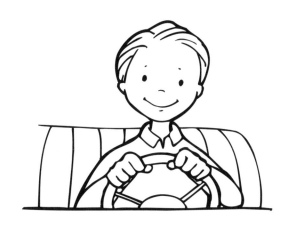

drive

© 1997 Super Duper® Publications 1-800-277-8737

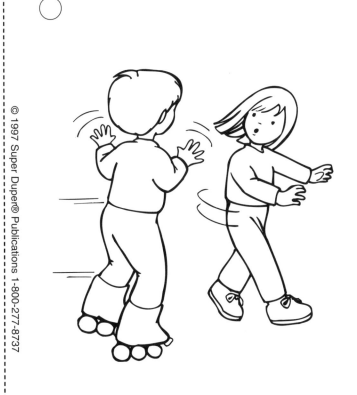

move

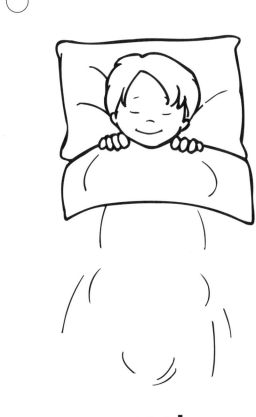

rest

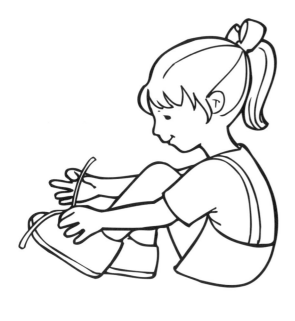

tie

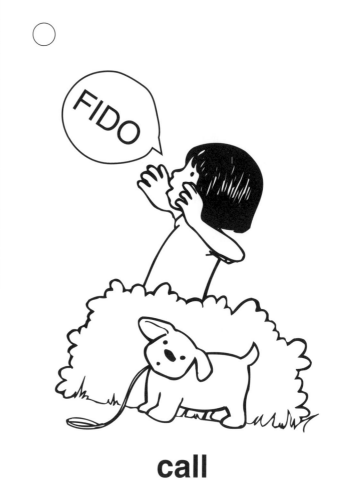

call

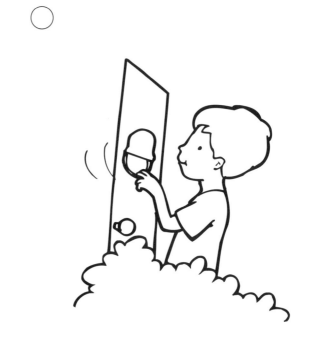

bring

knock

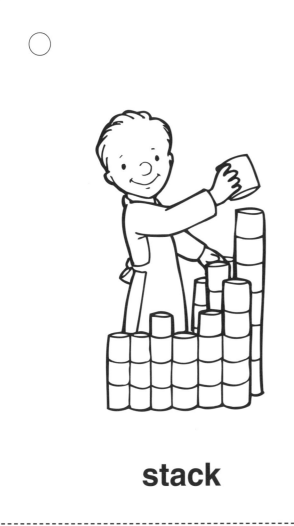

stack

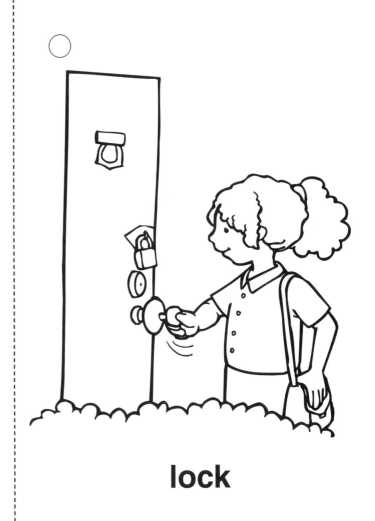

lock

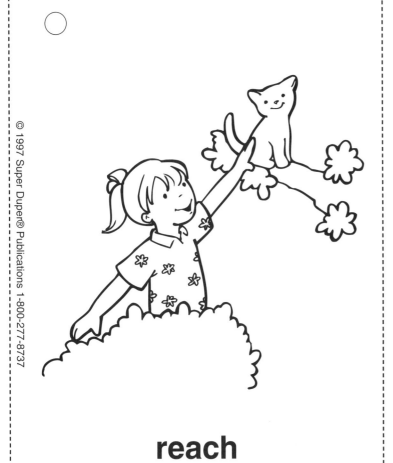

reach

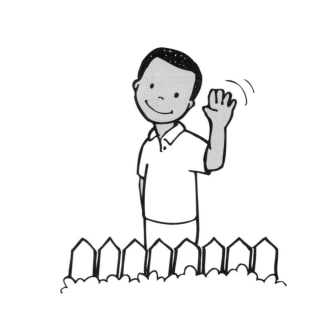

wave

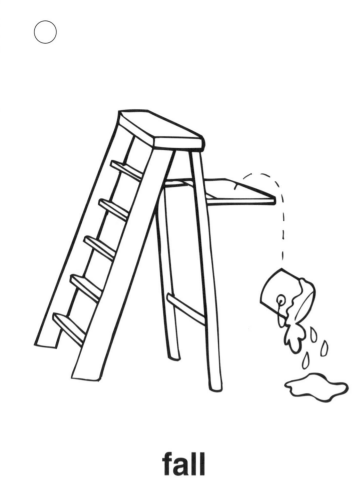

fall

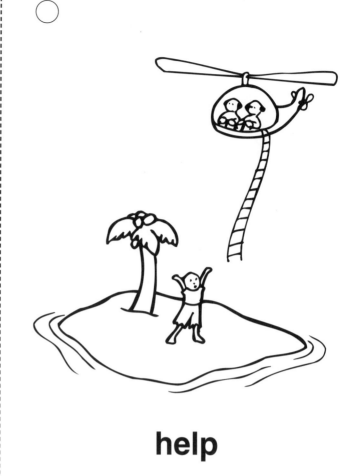

help

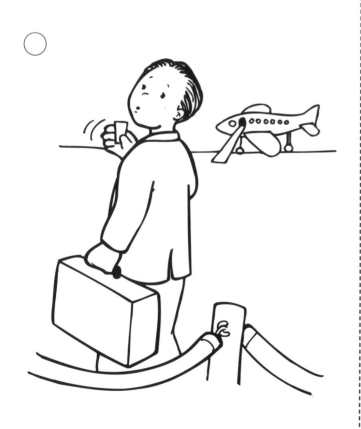

leave

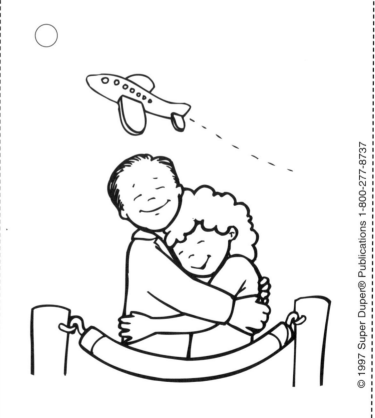

stay

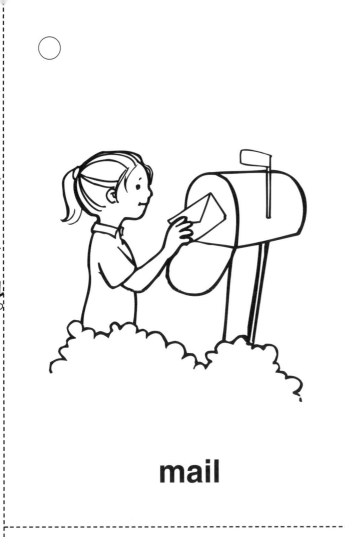

mail

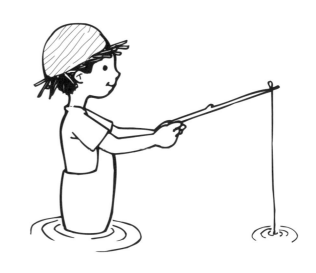

fish

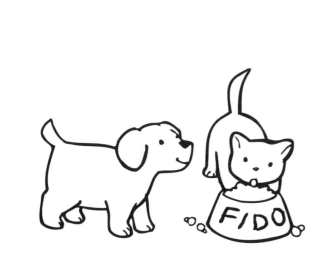

watch

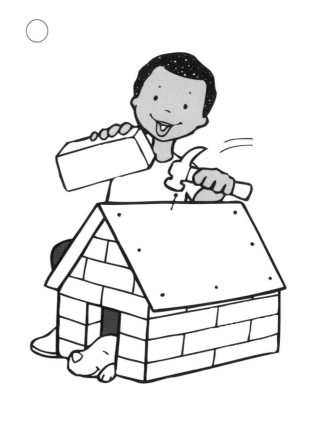

build

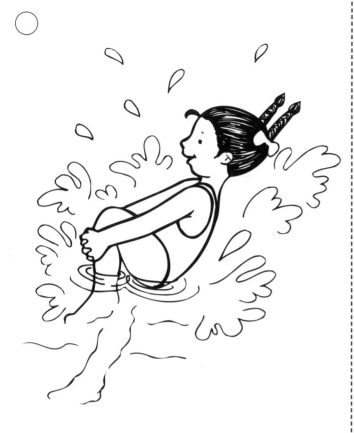

splash

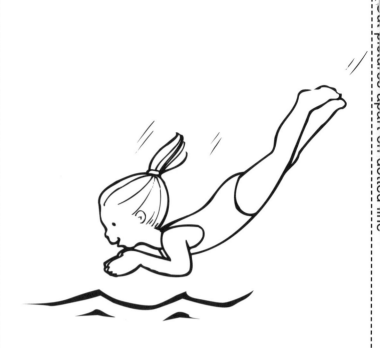

dive

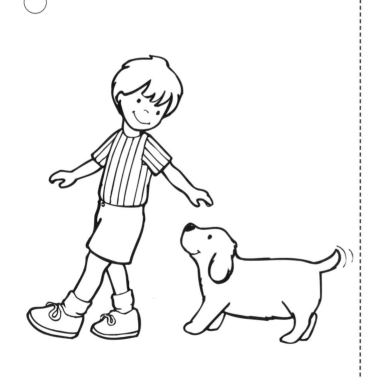

follow

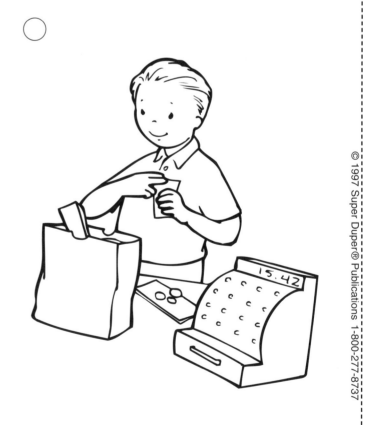

pay

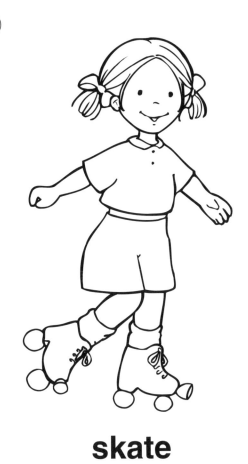

skate

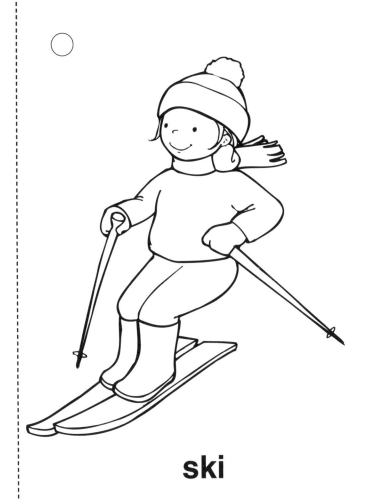

ski

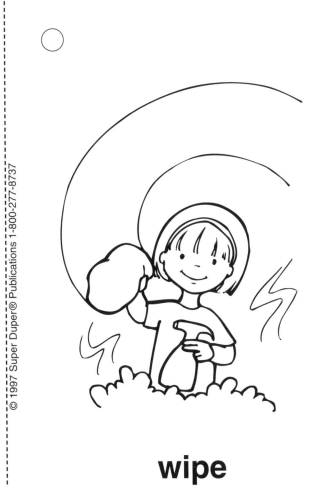

wipe

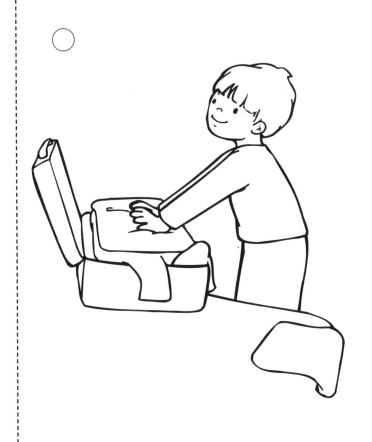

pack

65

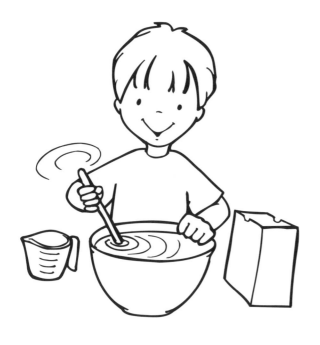

mix

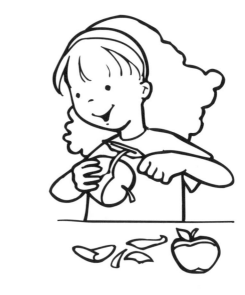

peel

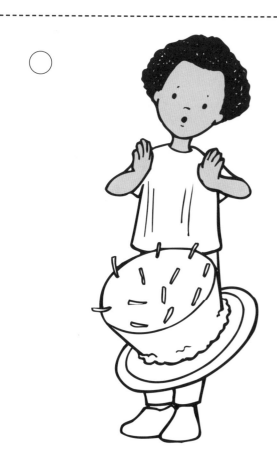

drop

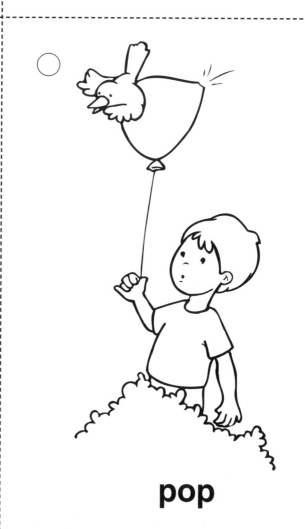

pop

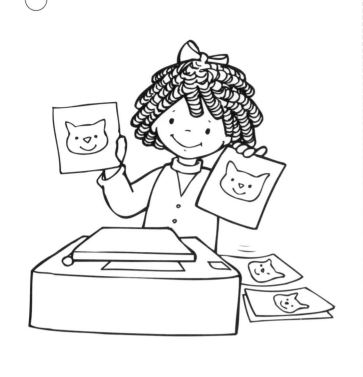

copy

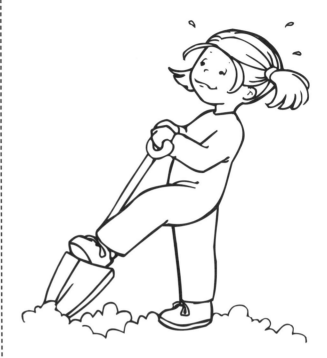

dig

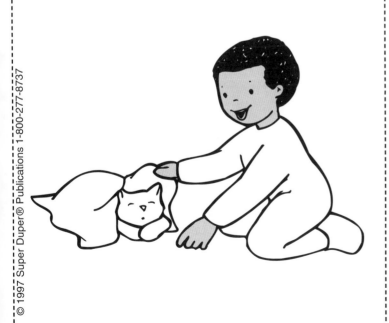

find

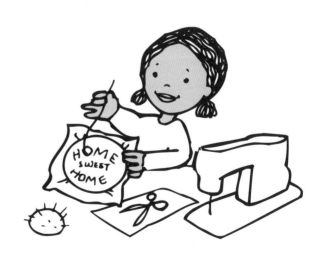

sew

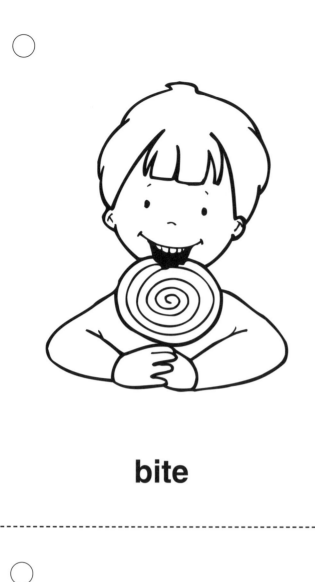

bite

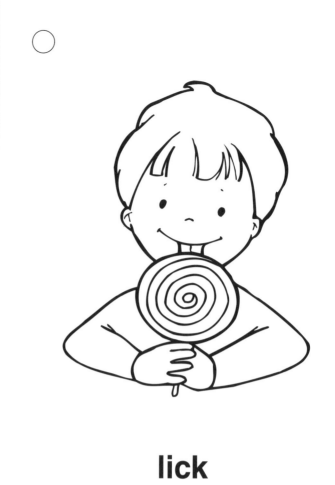

lick

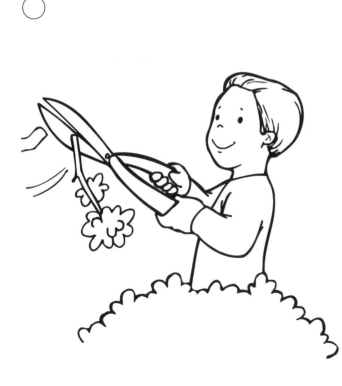

chop

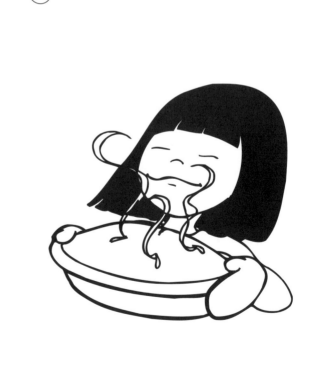

smell

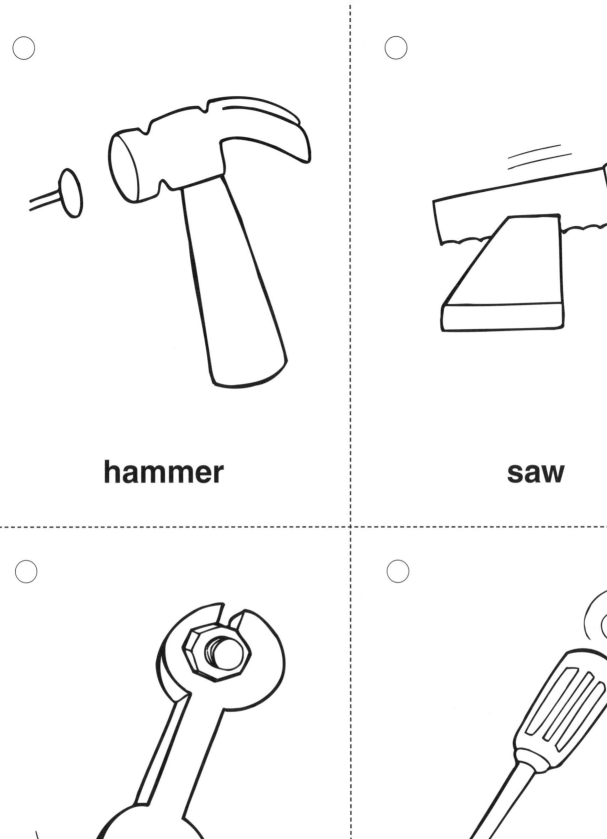

hammer

saw

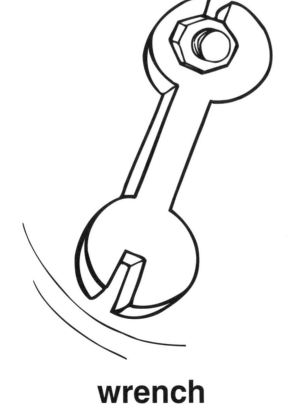

wrench

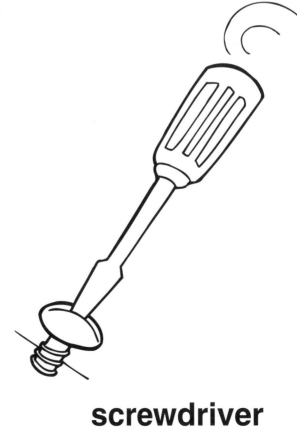

screwdriver

pliers

axe

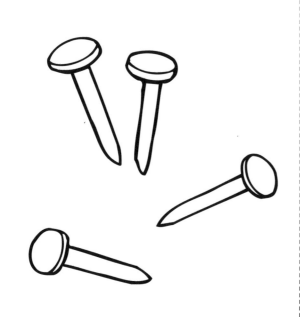

nails

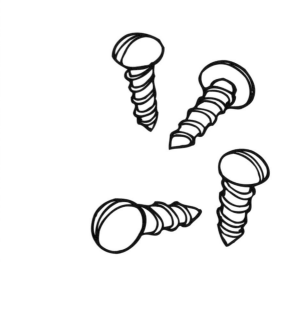

screws

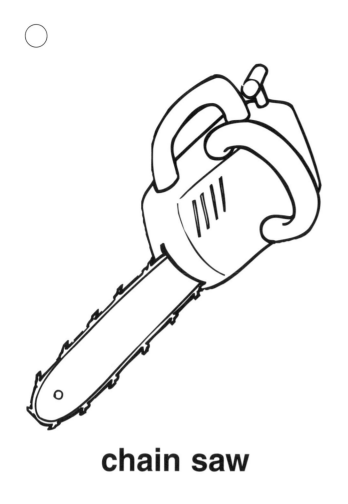

chain saw

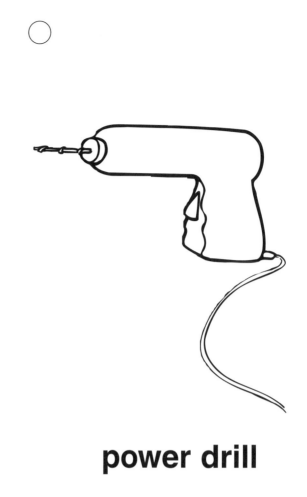

power drill

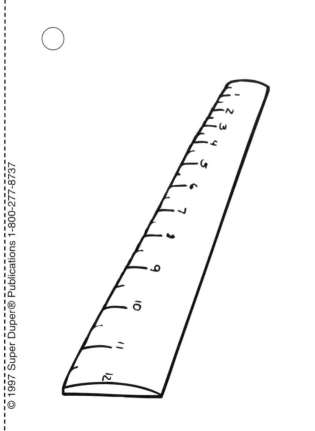

ruler

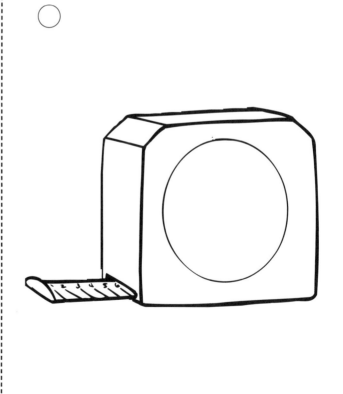

tape measure

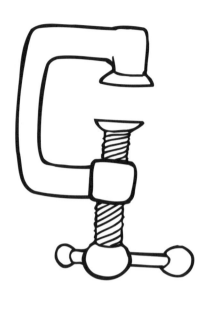

vise

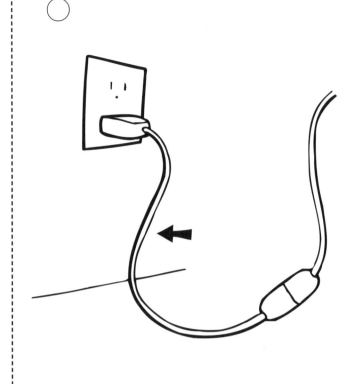

extension cord

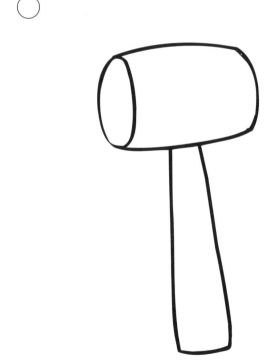

mallet

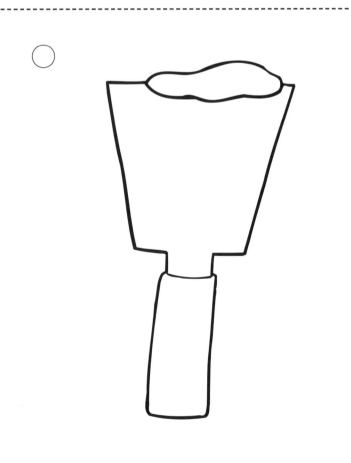

scraper/putty knife

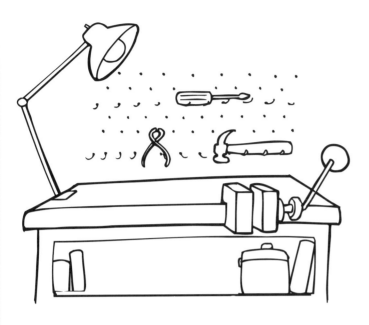

workbench

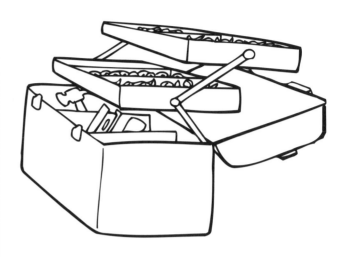

toolbox

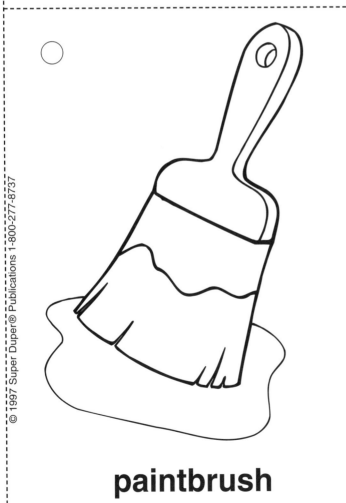

paintbrush

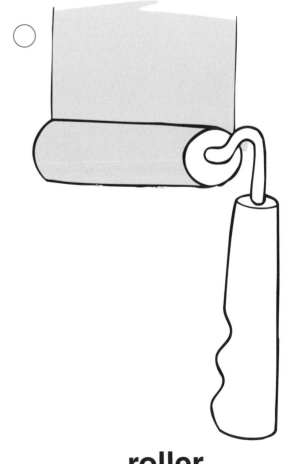

roller

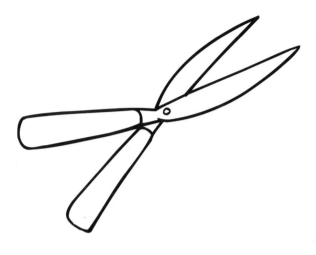

clippers

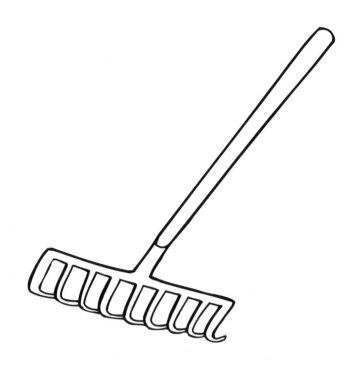

rake

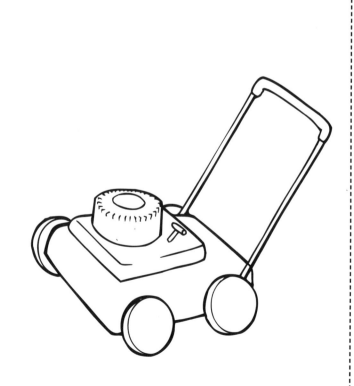

lawn mower

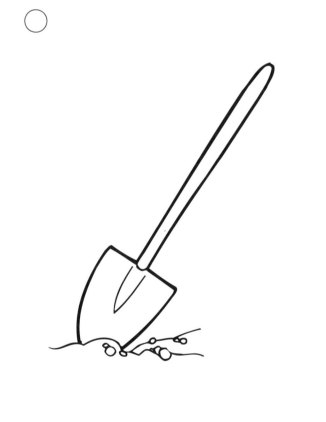

shovel

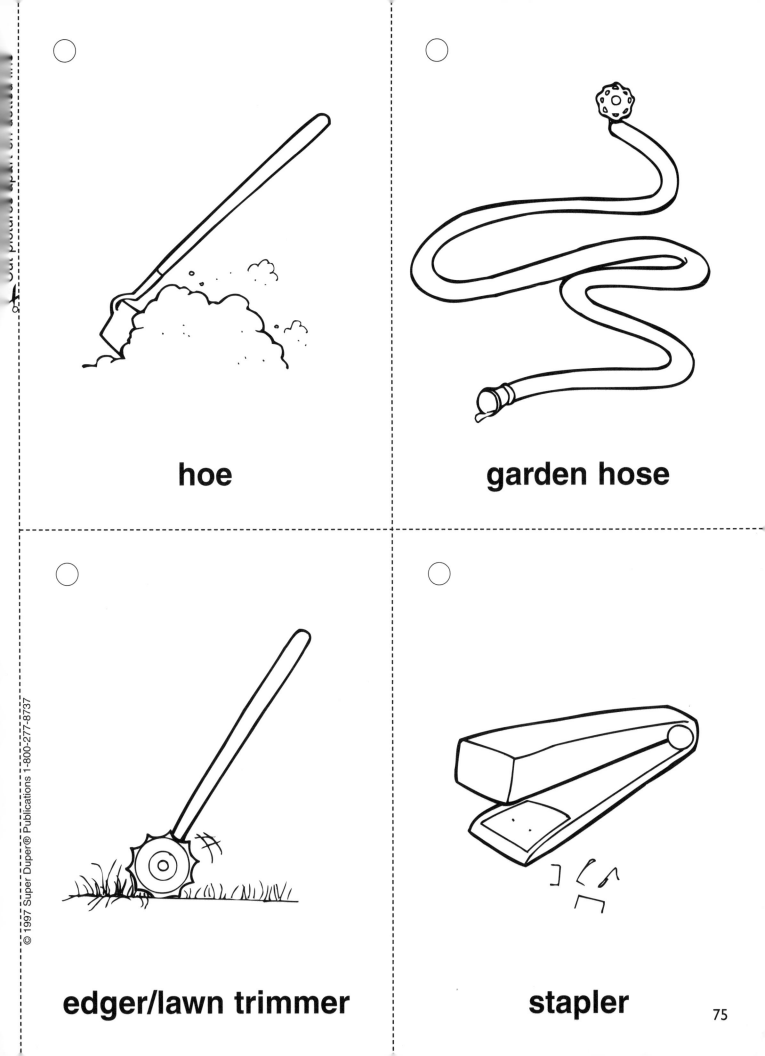

hoe

garden hose

edger/lawn trimmer

stapler

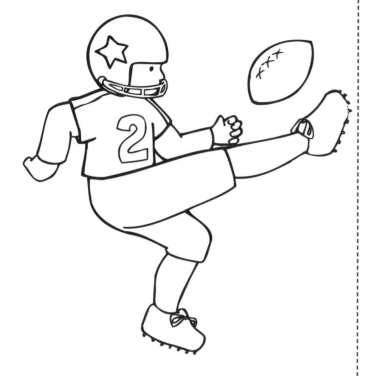

football

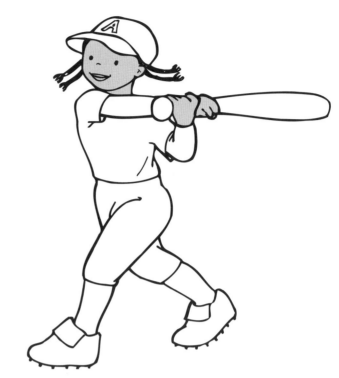

baseball

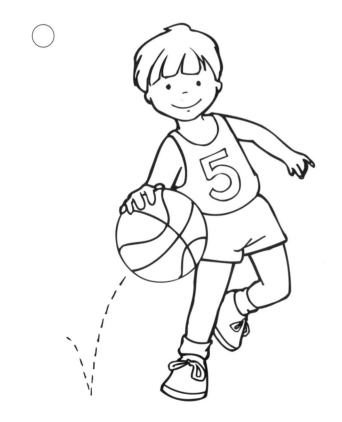

basketball

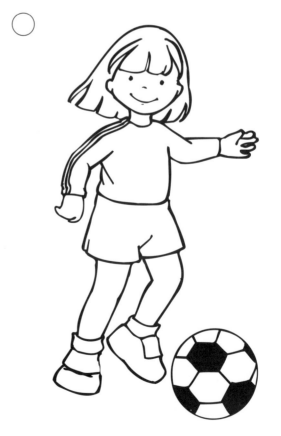

soccer

golf

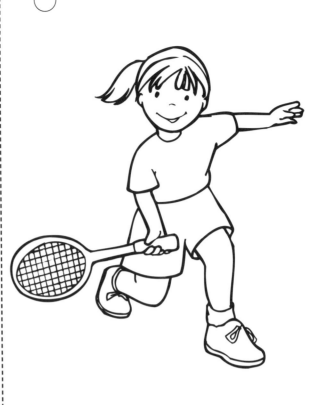

tennis

ice skating

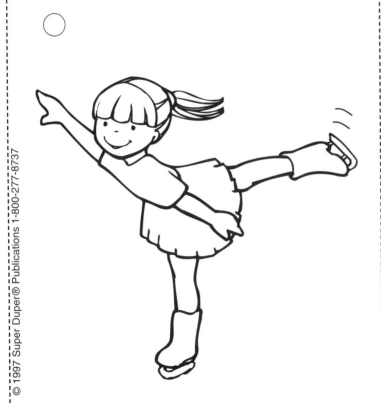

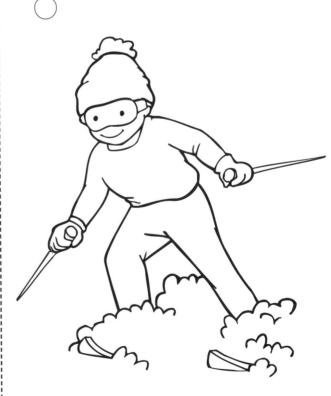

snow skiing

77

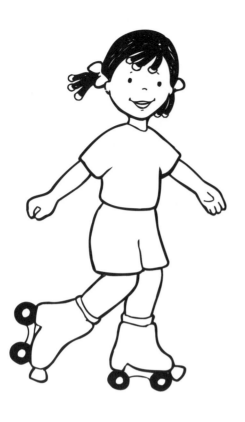

rollerskating

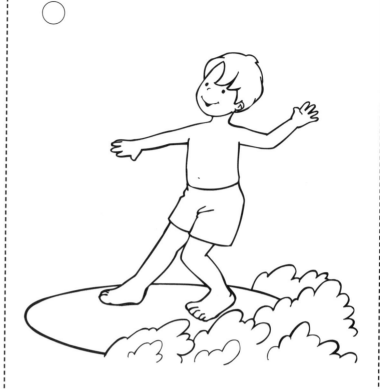

surfing

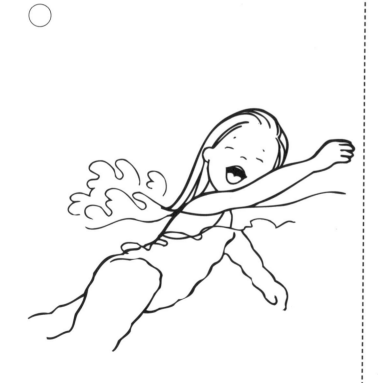

swimming

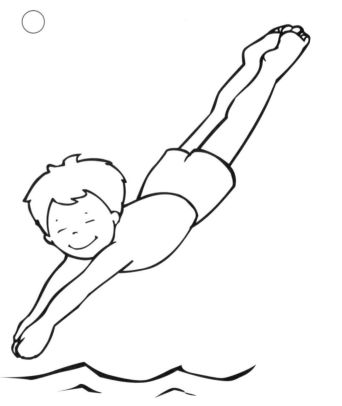

diving

78

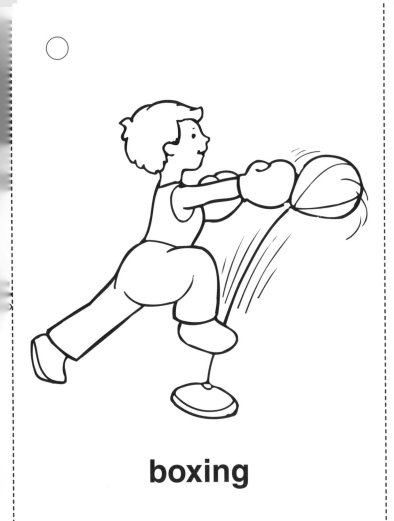

boxing

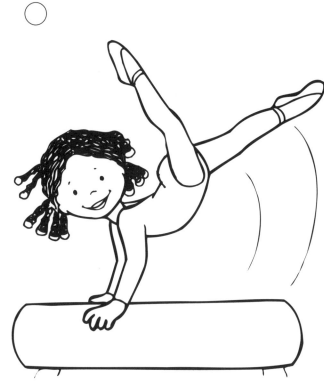

gymnastics

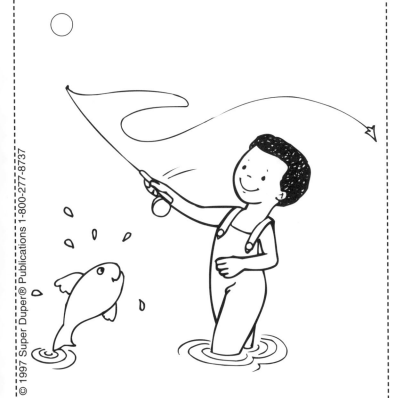

fishing

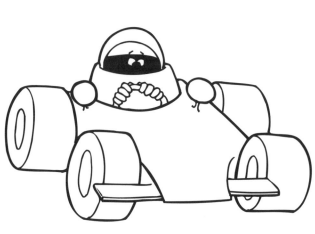

auto racing

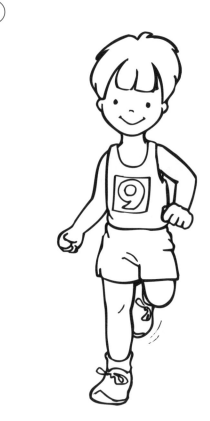

running/track

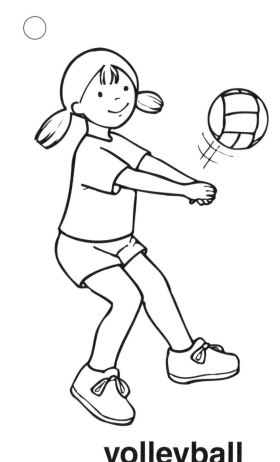

volleyball

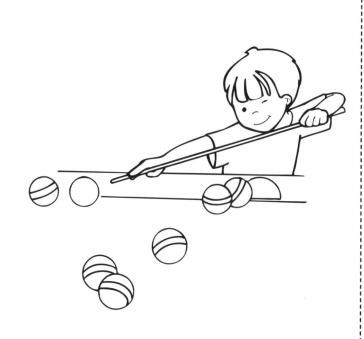

pool

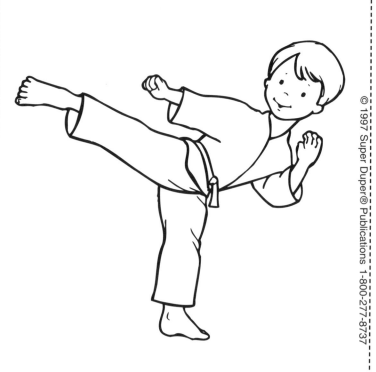

karate

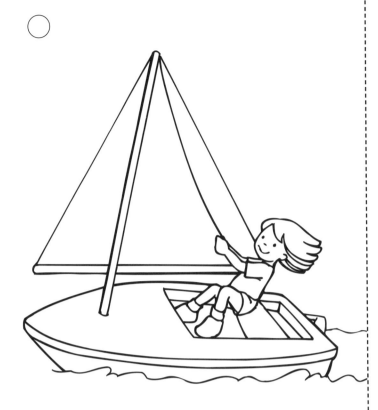

sailing

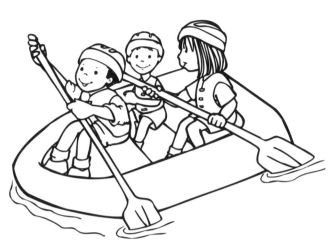

rafting

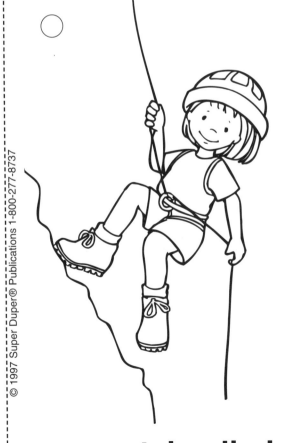

mountain climbing

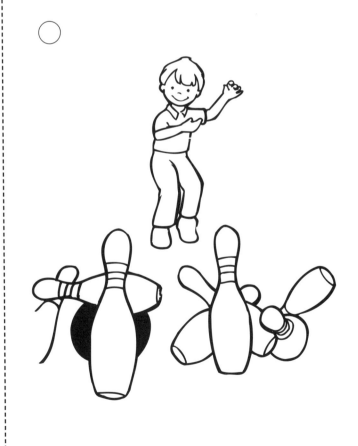

bowling

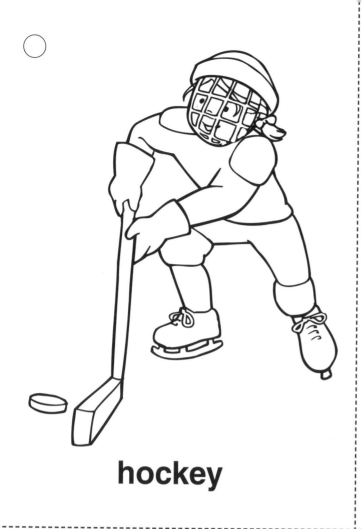

hockey

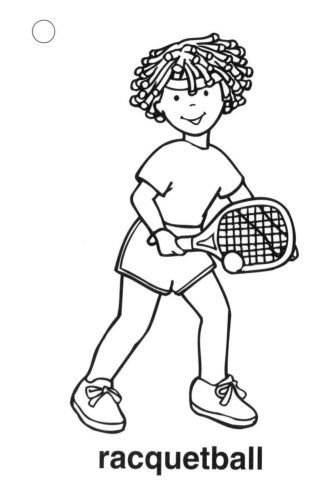

racquetball

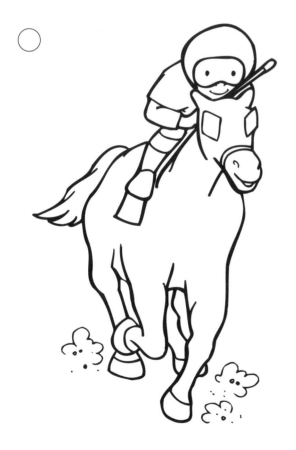

horse racing

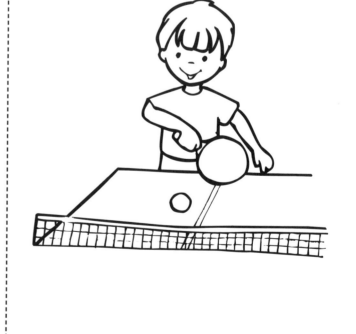

ping-pong

82

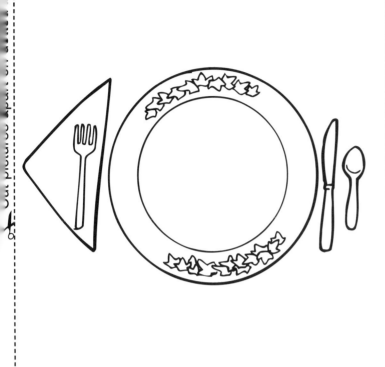

plate

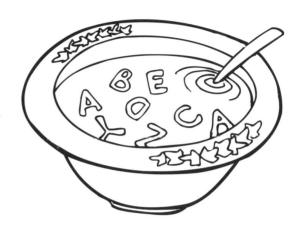

bowl

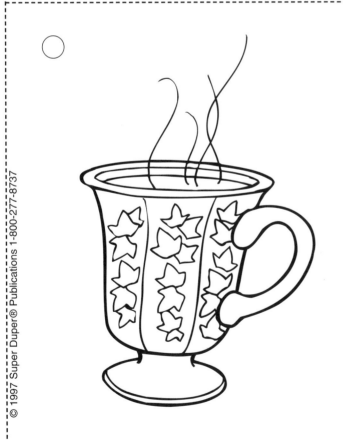

cup

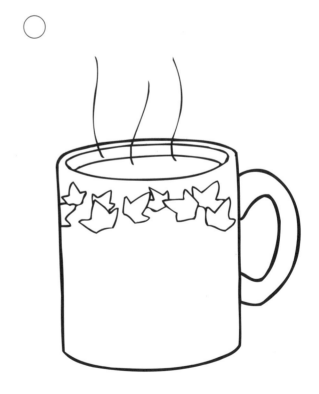

mug

83

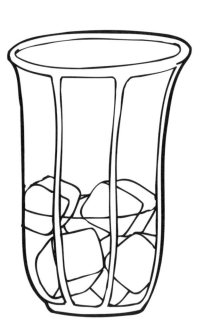

glass

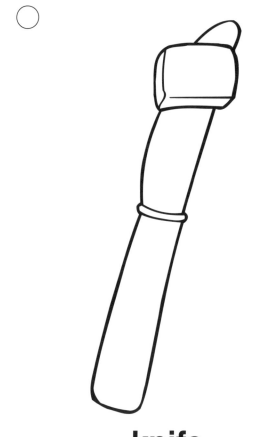

knife

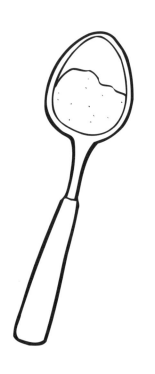

spoon

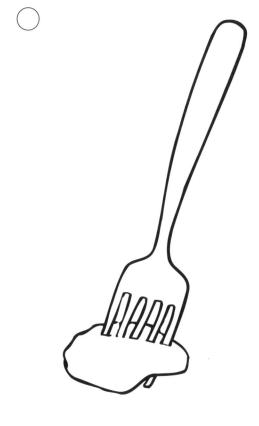

fork

Cut pictures apart on dotted line

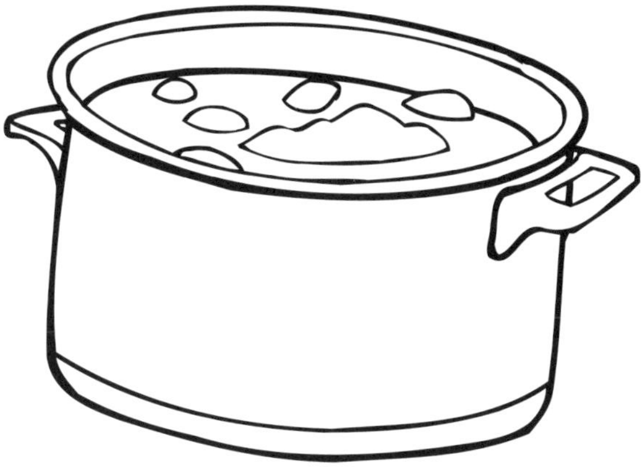

pot

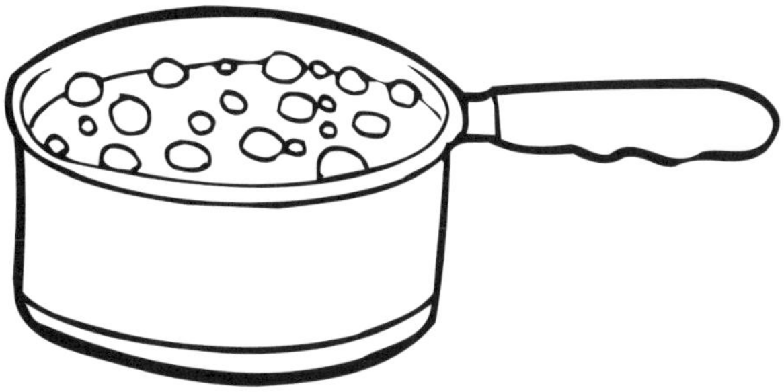

saucepan

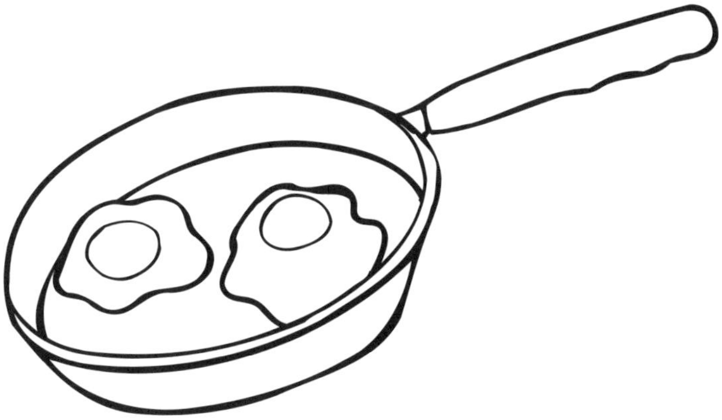

skillet or frying pan

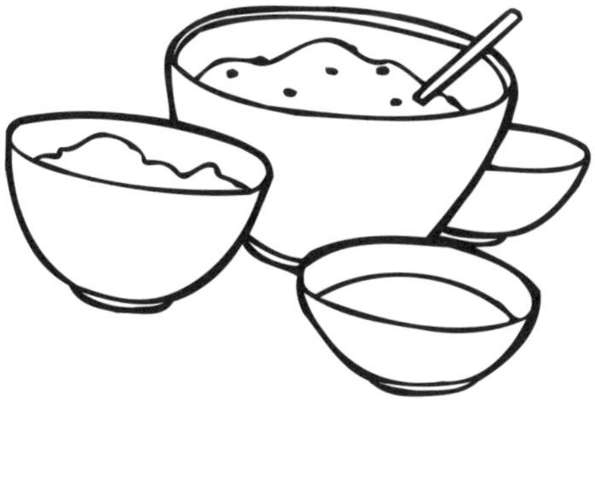

mixing bowls

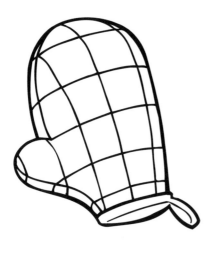

pot holder

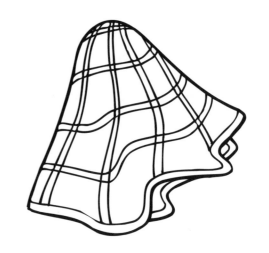

dishrag/dishcloth

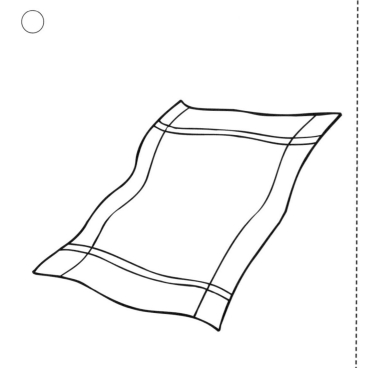

towel

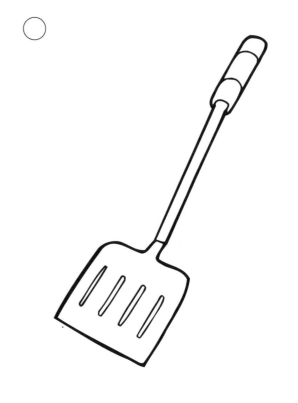

spatula

napkin

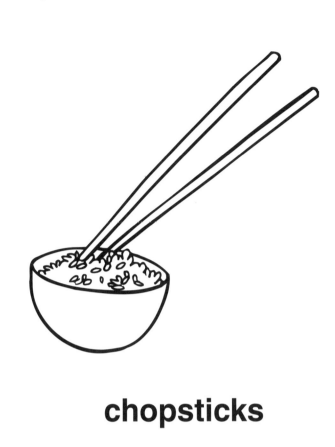

chopsticks

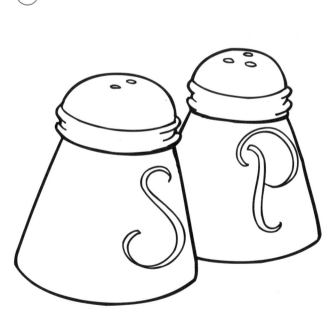

salt & pepper shakers

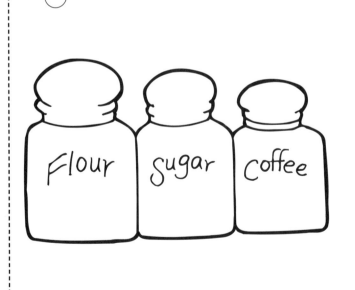

Flour   sugar   coffee

canisters

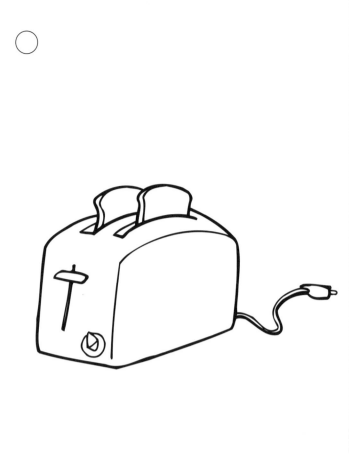

toaster

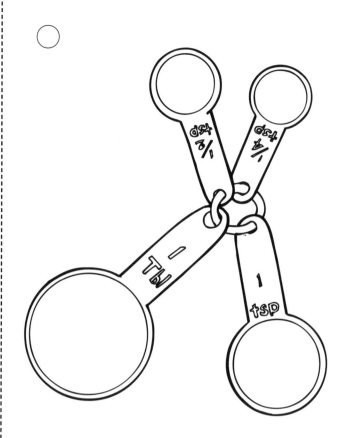

measuring spoons

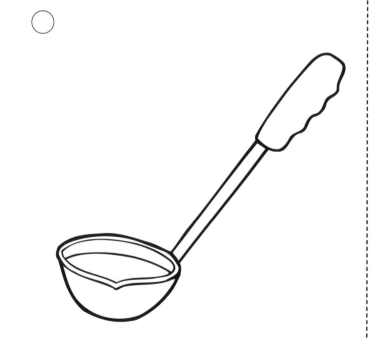

ladle

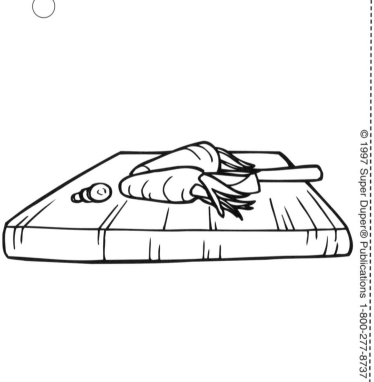

cutting board

rolling pin

tea kettle

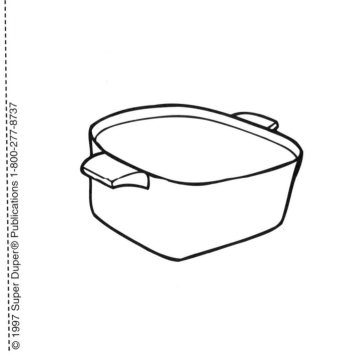

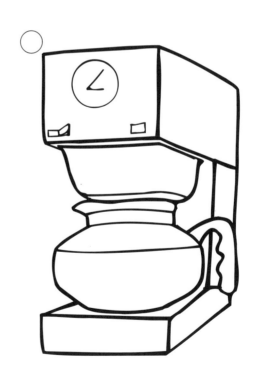

casserole dish

coffee maker

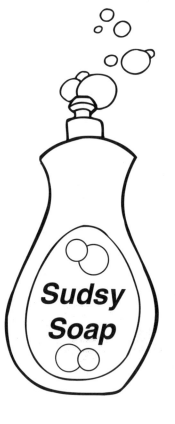

dish soap

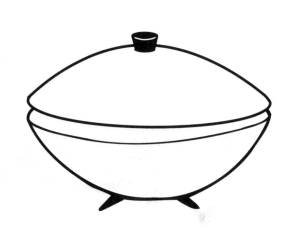

wok

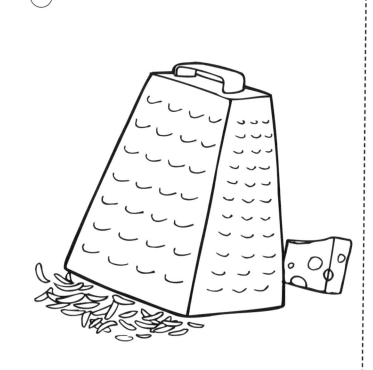

grater

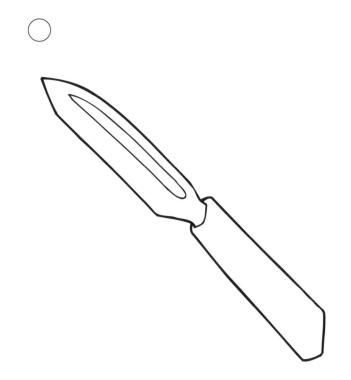

vegetable peeler

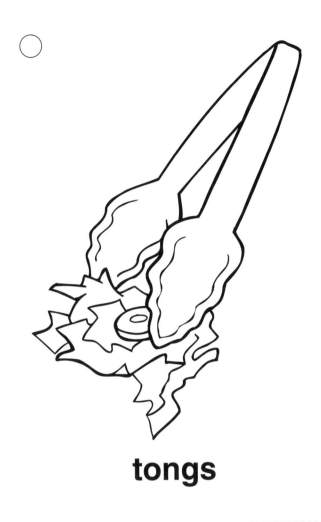

tongs

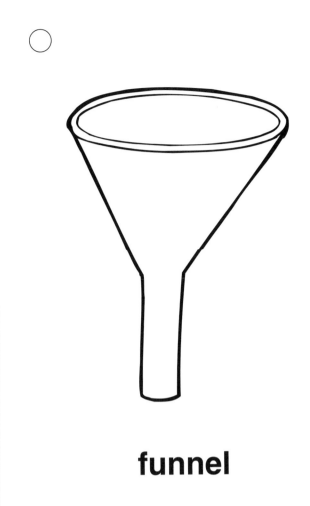

funnel

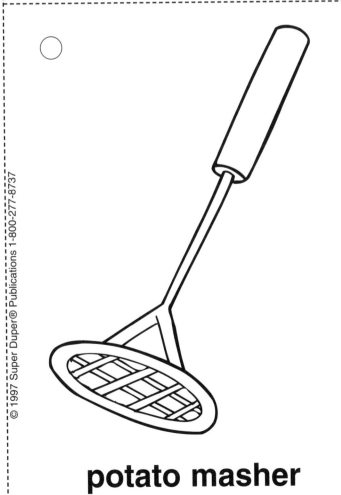

potato masher

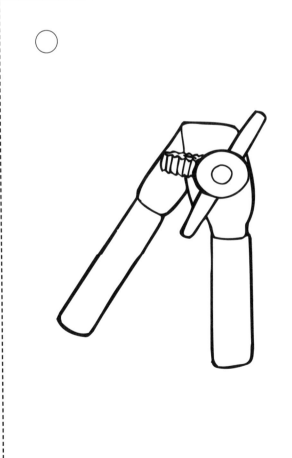

can opener

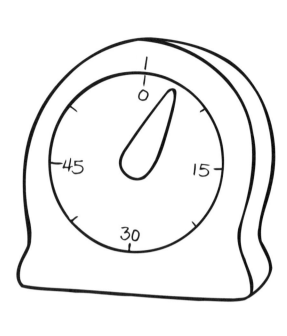

timer

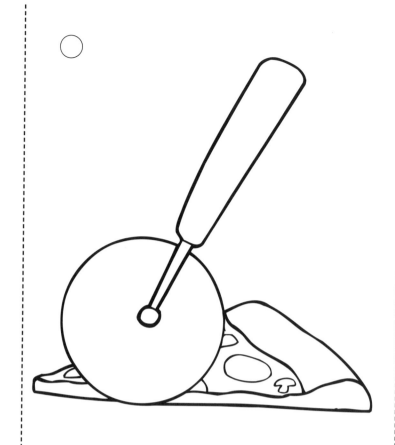

pizza cutter

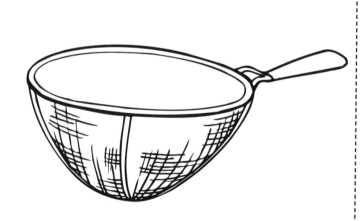

strainer

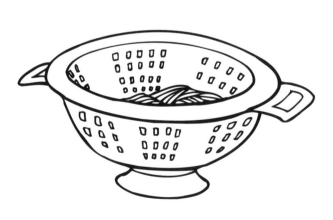

colander

© 1997 Super Duper® Publications 1-800-277-8737

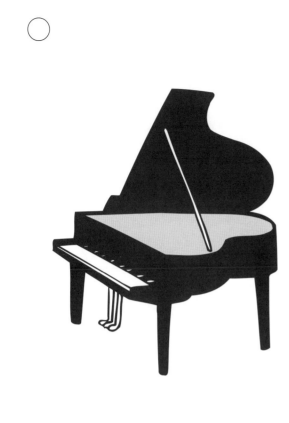

piano

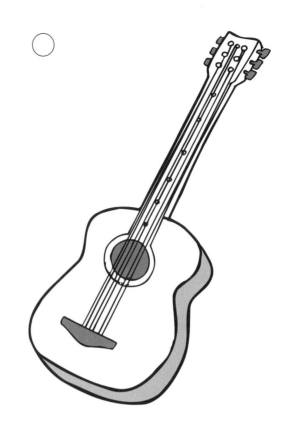

guitar

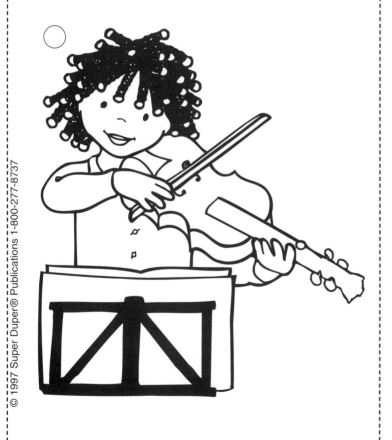

violin

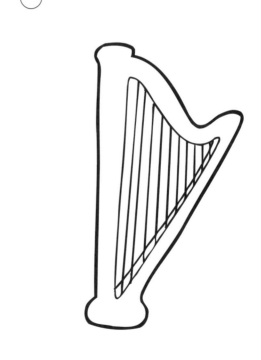

harp

93

banjo

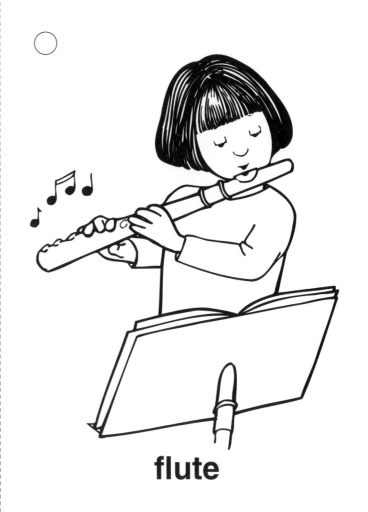

flute

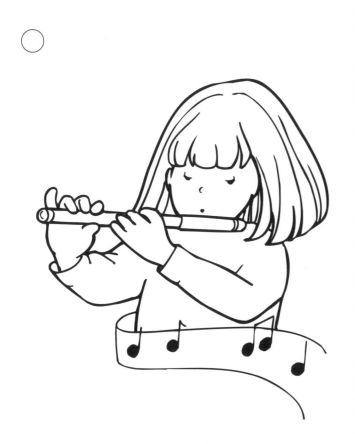

piccolo

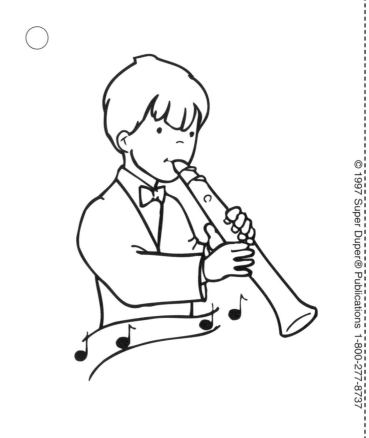

clarinet

© 1997 Super Duper® Publications 1-800-277-8737

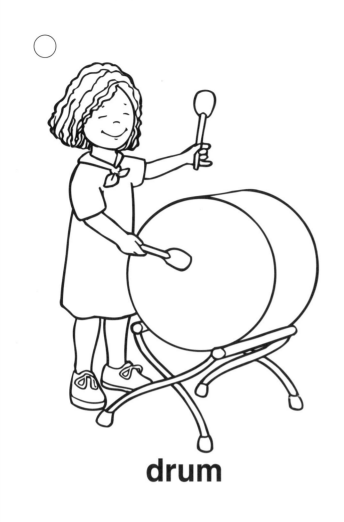

drum

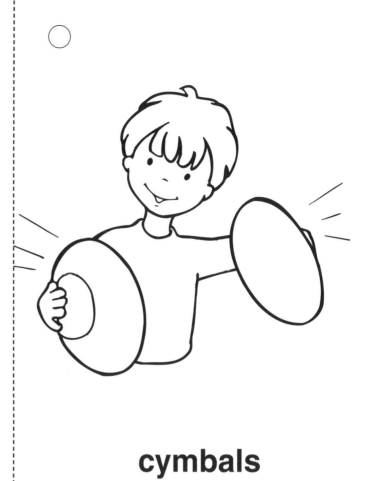

cymbals

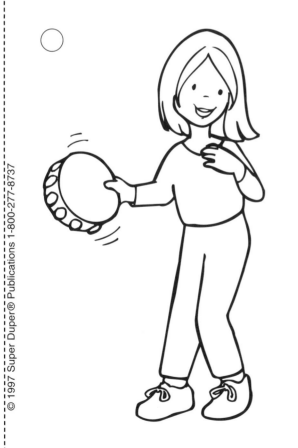

tambourine

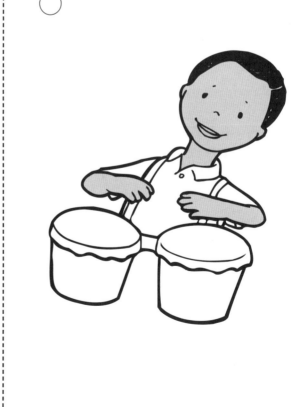

bongos

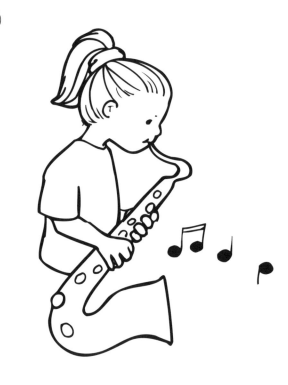

saxophone

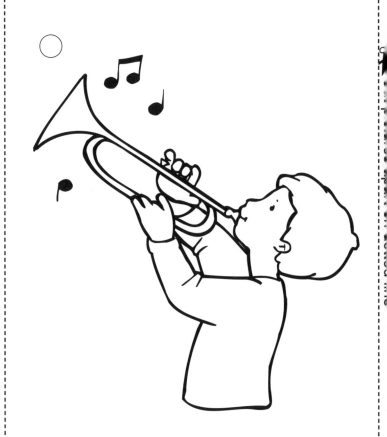

trumpet

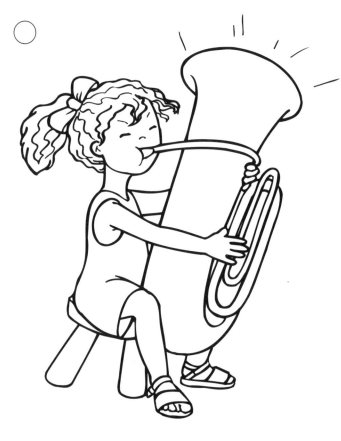

tuba

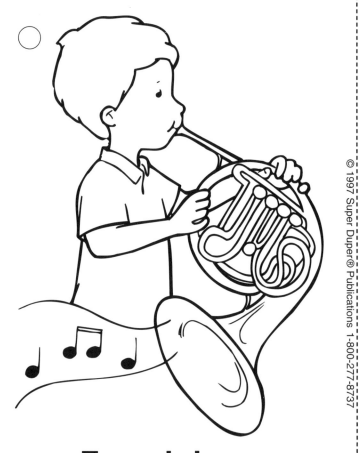

French horn

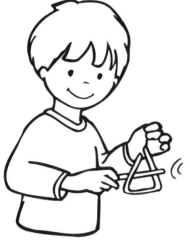

triangle

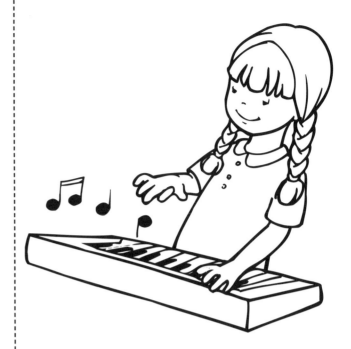

keyboard

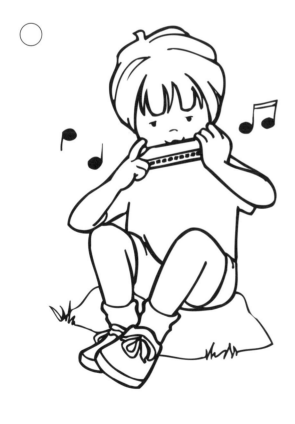

harmonica

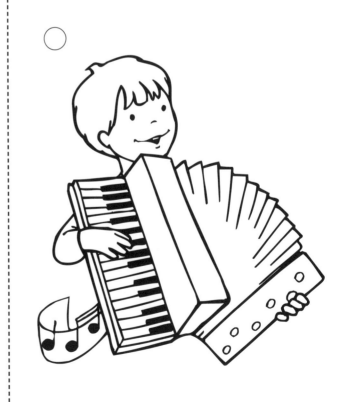

accordion

97

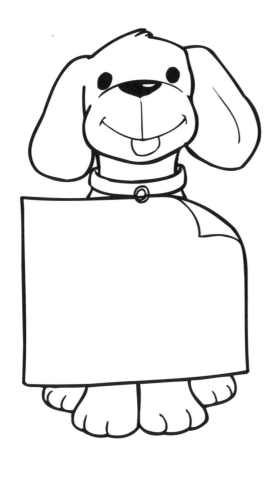
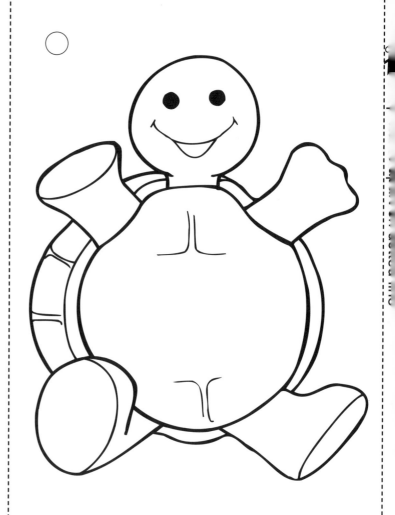

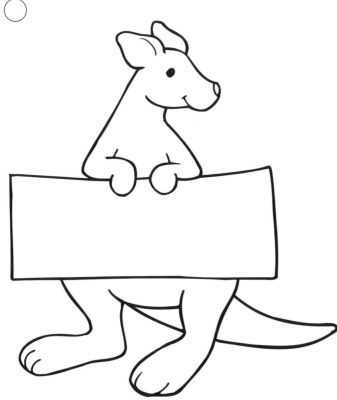
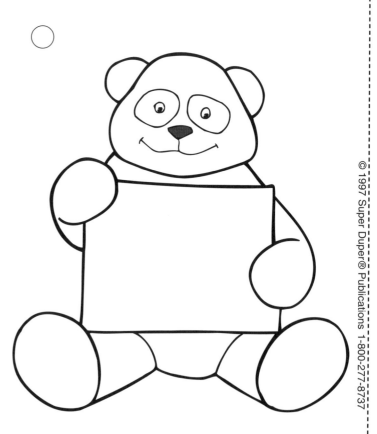

98

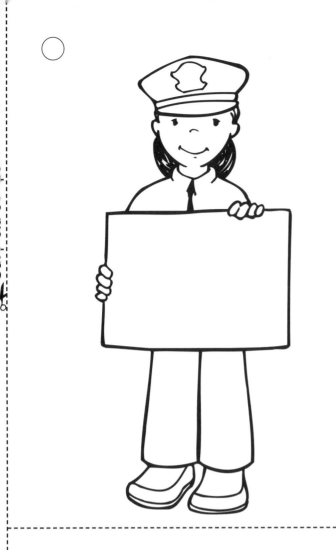

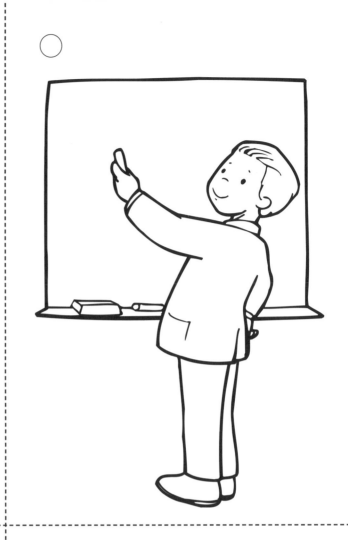

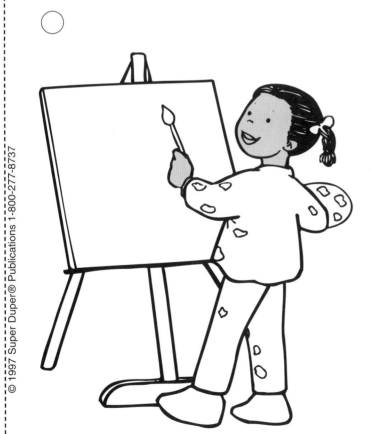

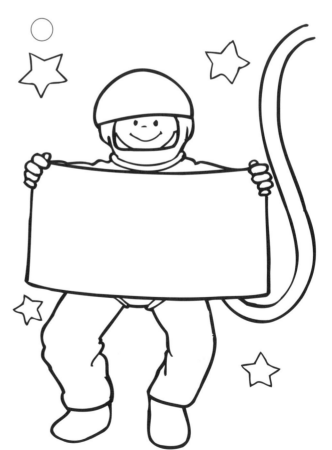

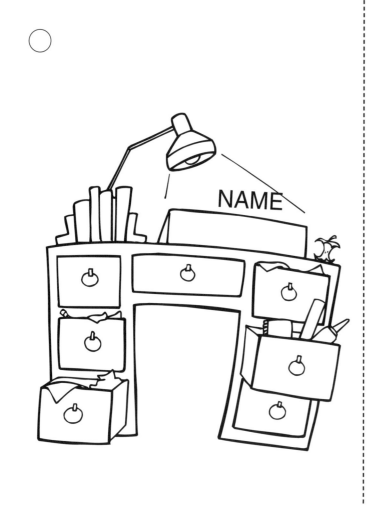

NAME

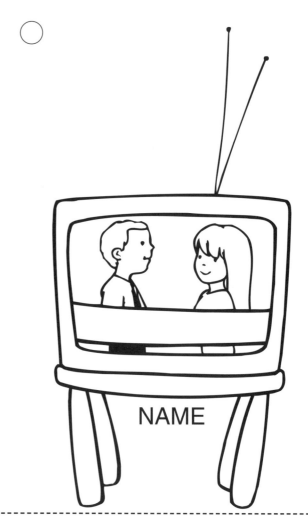

NAME

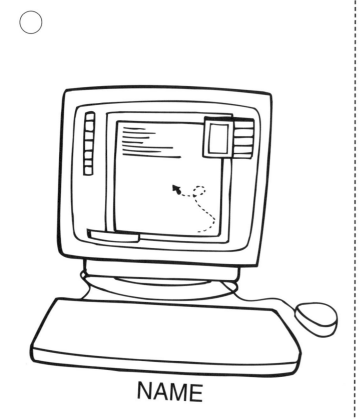

NAME

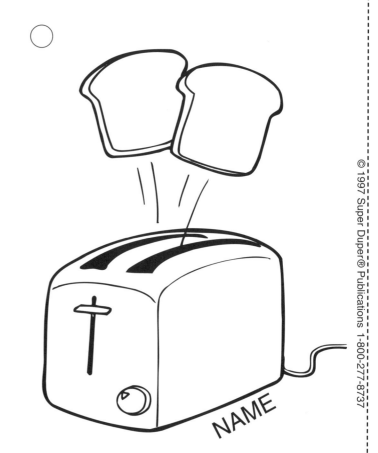

NAME

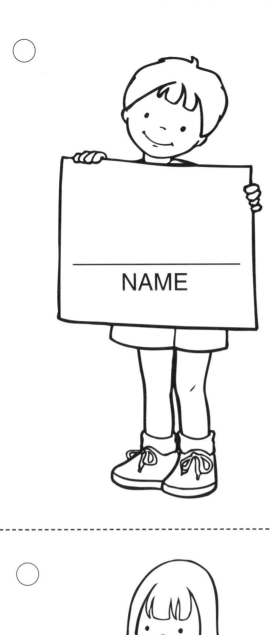

NAME

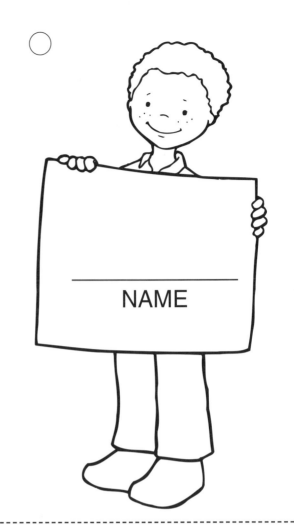

NAME

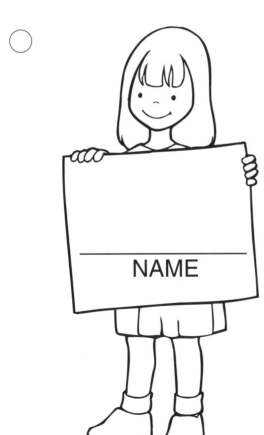

NAME

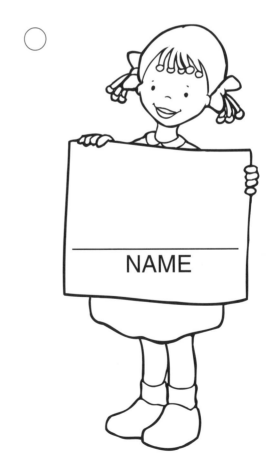

NAME

_____
NAME

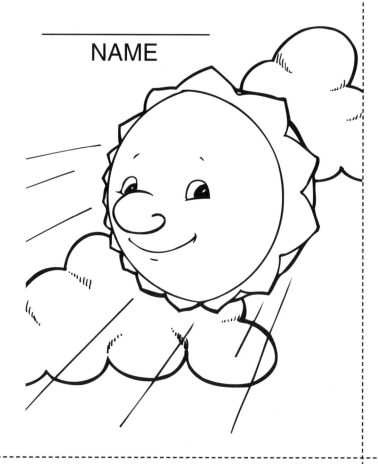

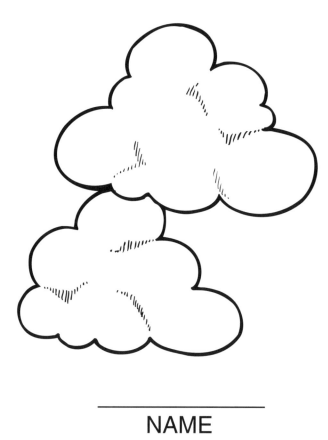

_____
NAME

_____
NAME

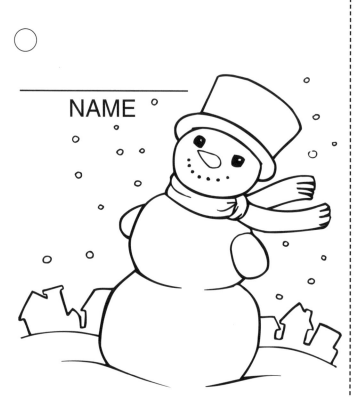

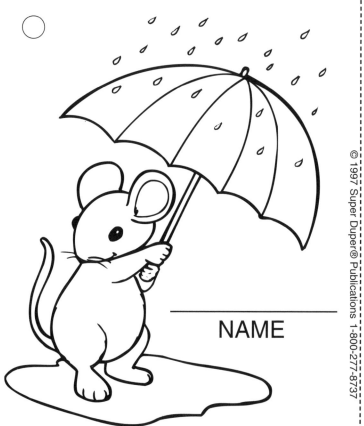

_____
NAME

102

© 1997 Super Duper® Publications 1-800-277-8737

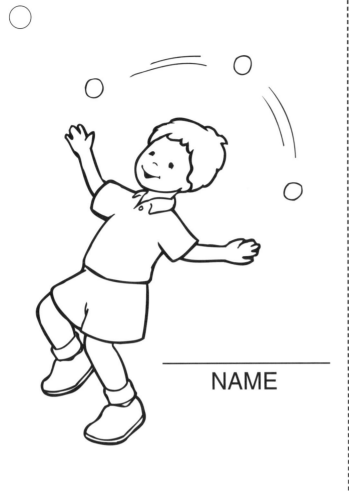

NAME

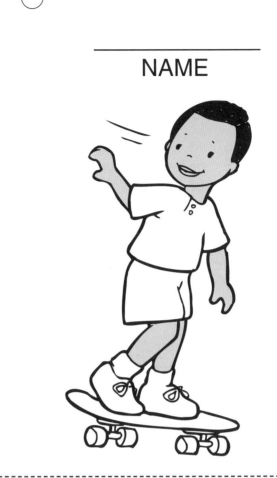

NAME

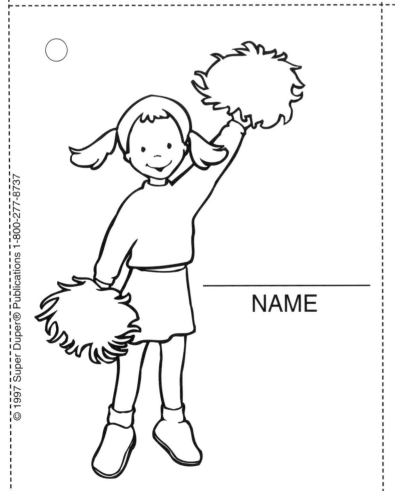

NAME

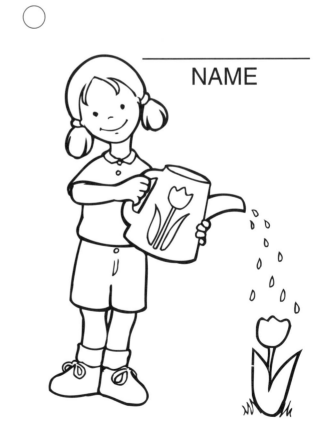

NAME

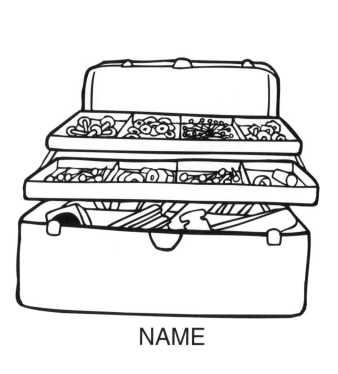

NAME

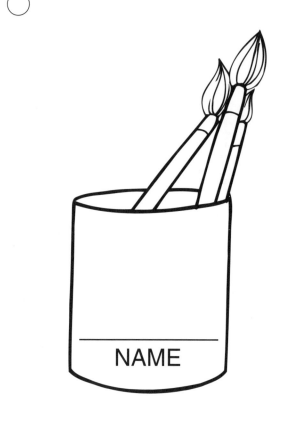

NAME

_____
NAME

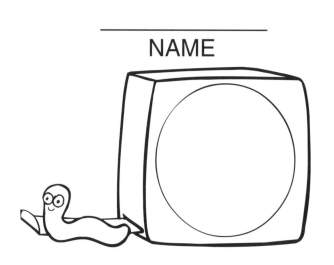

_____
NAME

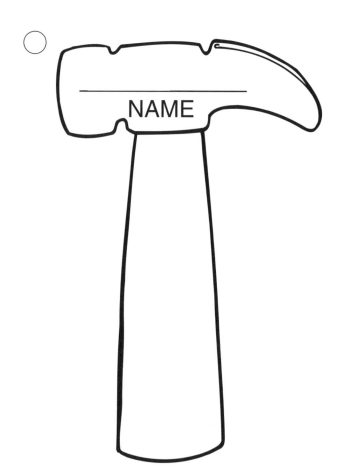

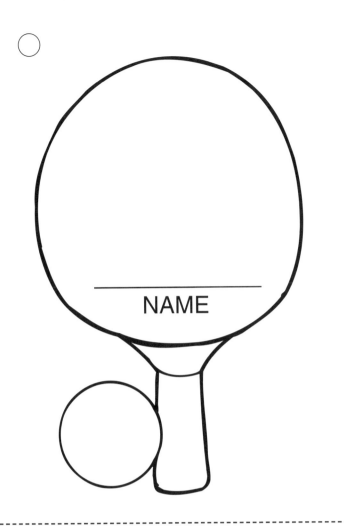

NAME

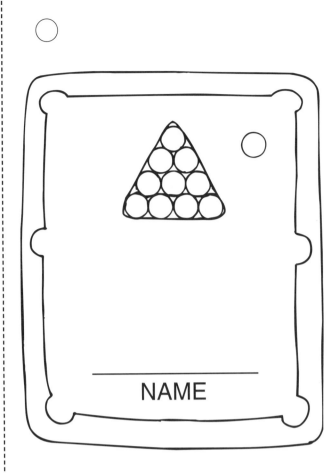

NAME

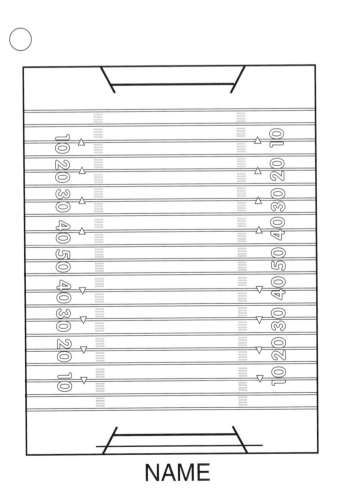

NAME

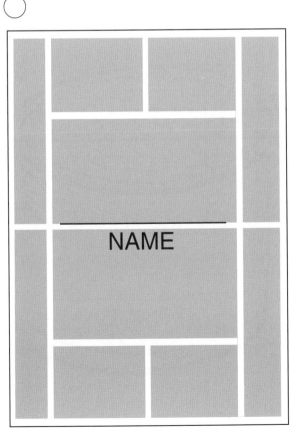

NAME

© 1997 Super Duper® Publications 1-800-277-8737

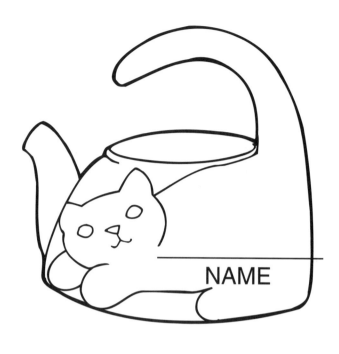

NAME

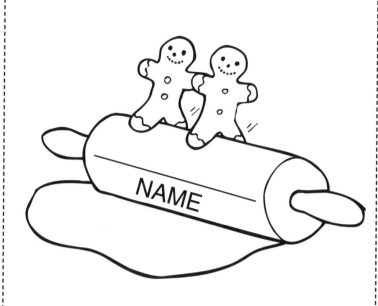

NAME

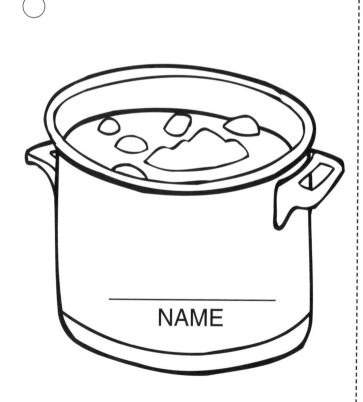

NAME

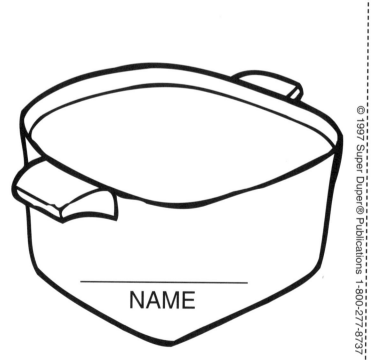

NAME

© 1997 Super Duper® Publications 1-800-277-8737

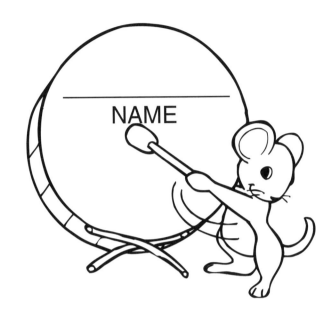

NAME

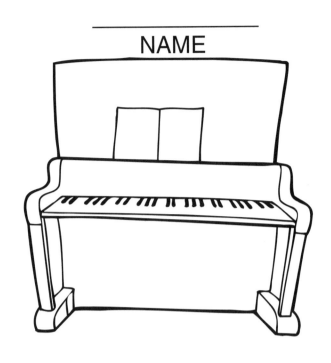

NAME

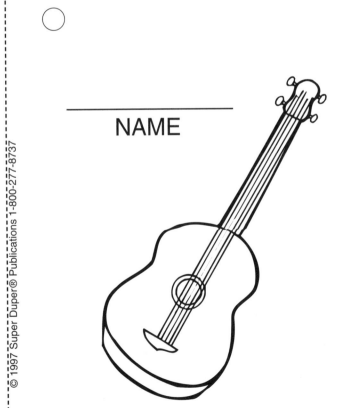

NAME

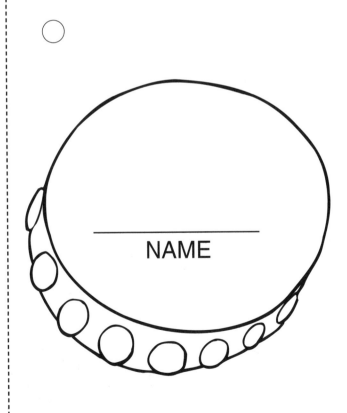

NAME

107

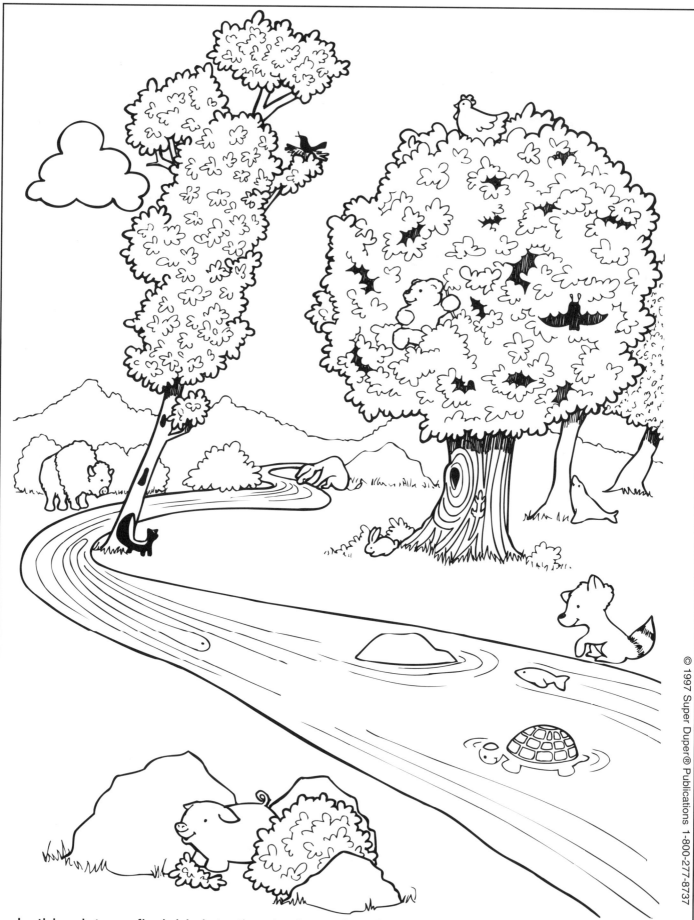

In this picture, find: bird, turtle, donkey, pig, chicken, rabbit, fox, fish, lizard, snake, bear, bison, bat, seal, and skunk.

108 Super Duper® Publications 1-800-277-8737

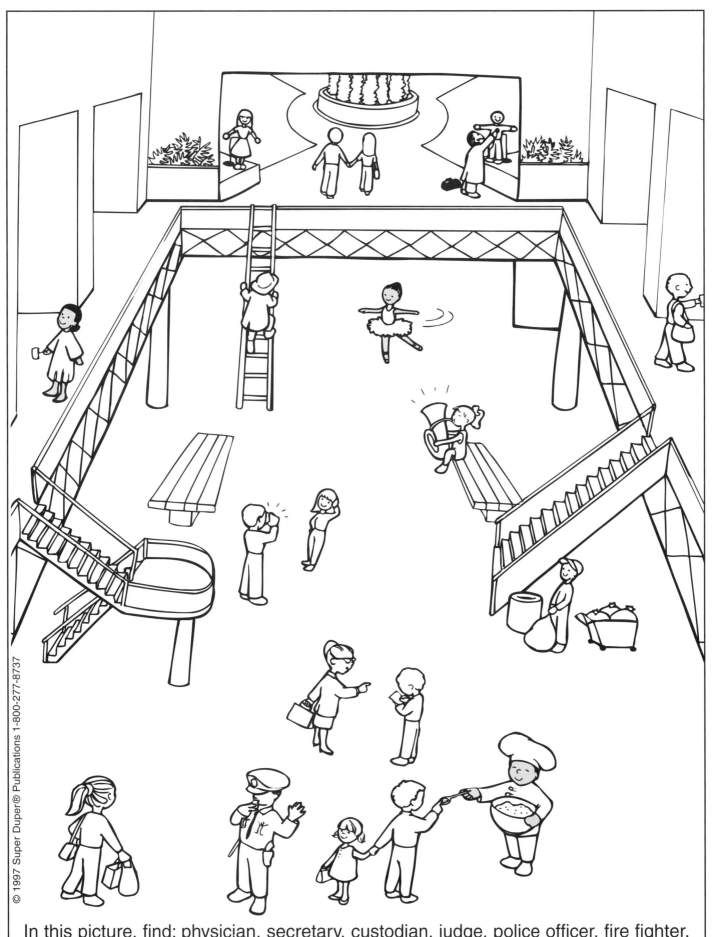

In this picture, find: physician, secretary, custodian, judge, police officer, fire fighter, dancer, chef, mail carrier, photographer, and musician.

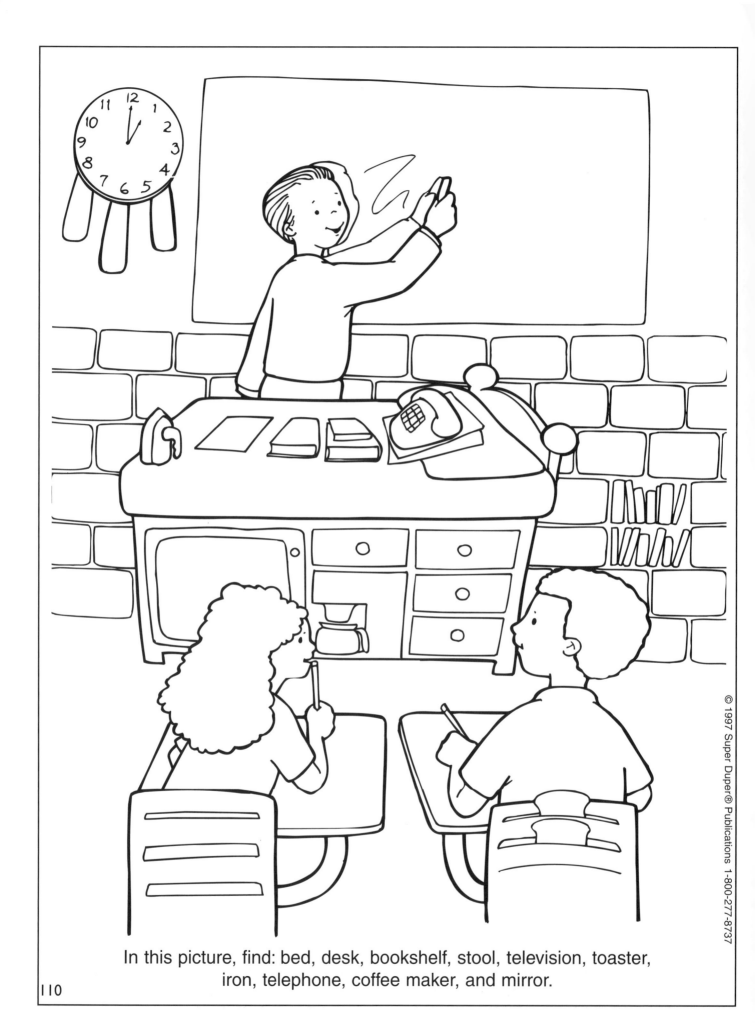

In this picture, find: bed, desk, bookshelf, stool, television, toaster, iron, telephone, coffee maker, and mirror.

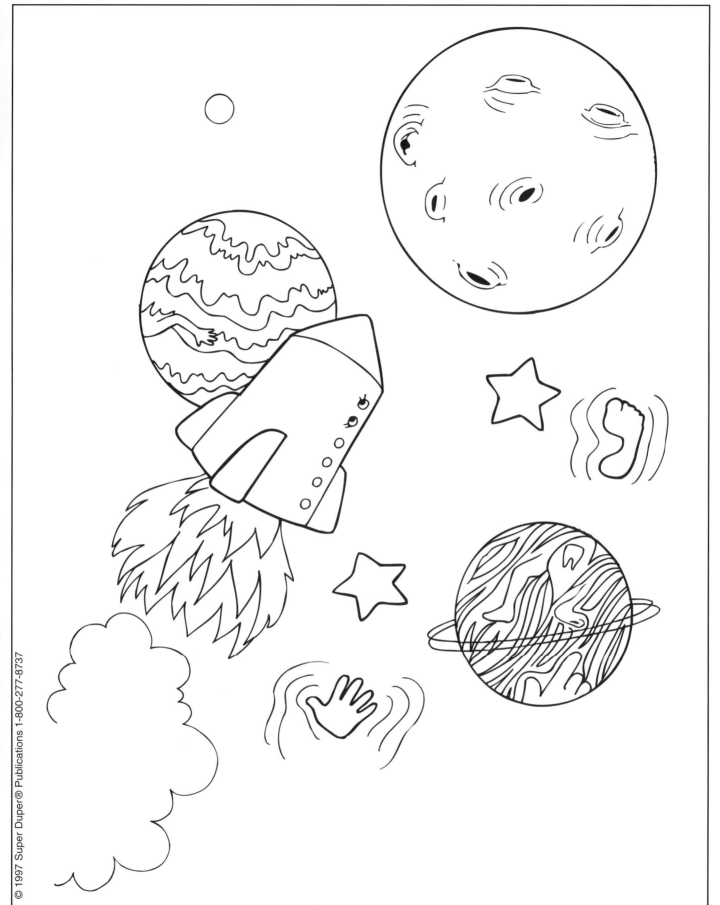

In this picture, find: eyes, ears, lips, nose, hand, tooth, finger, leg, and foot.

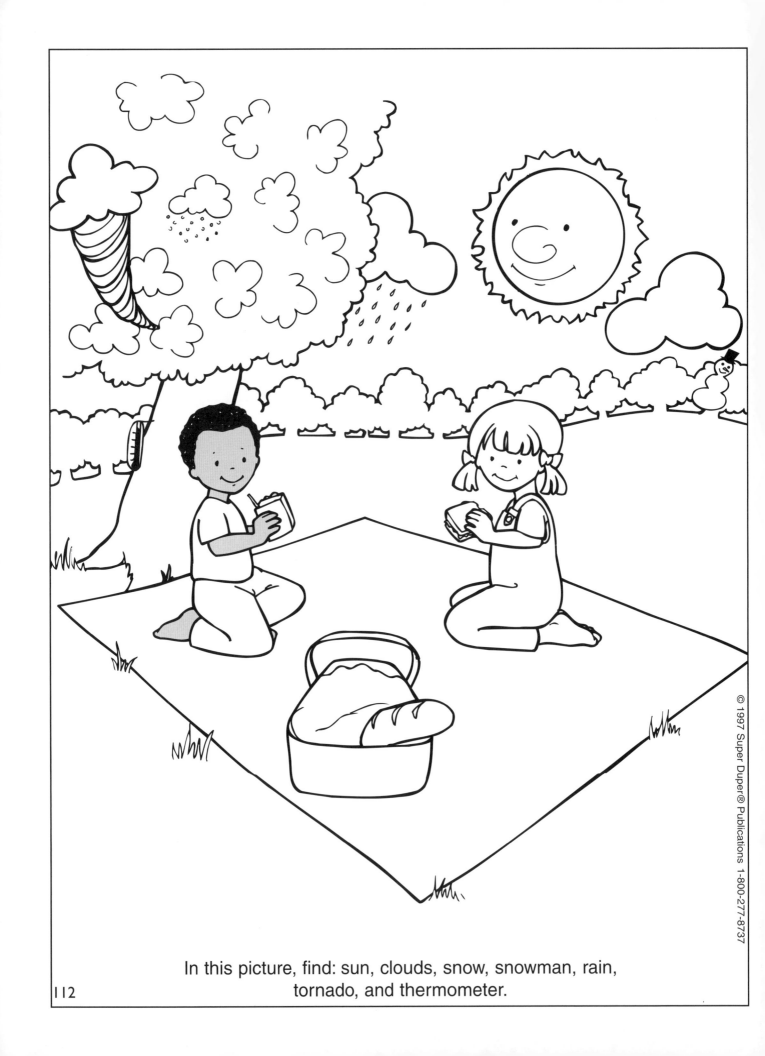

In this picture, find: sun, clouds, snow, snowman, rain, tornado, and thermometer.

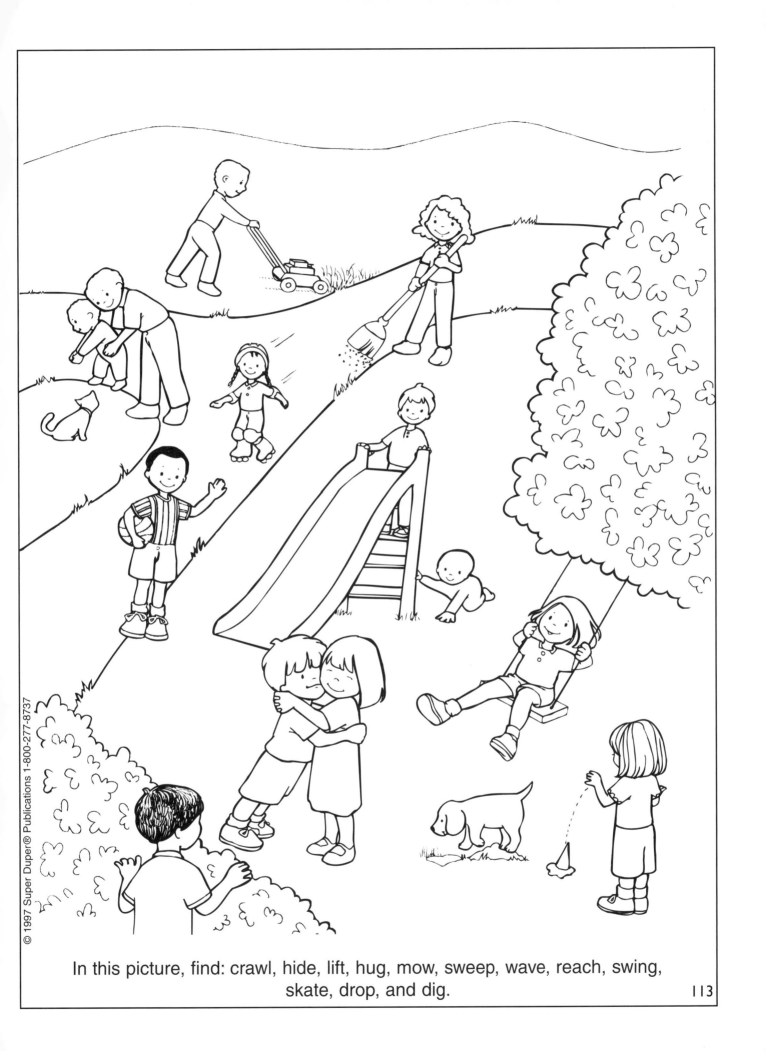

In this picture, find: crawl, hide, lift, hug, mow, sweep, wave, reach, swing, skate, drop, and dig.

113

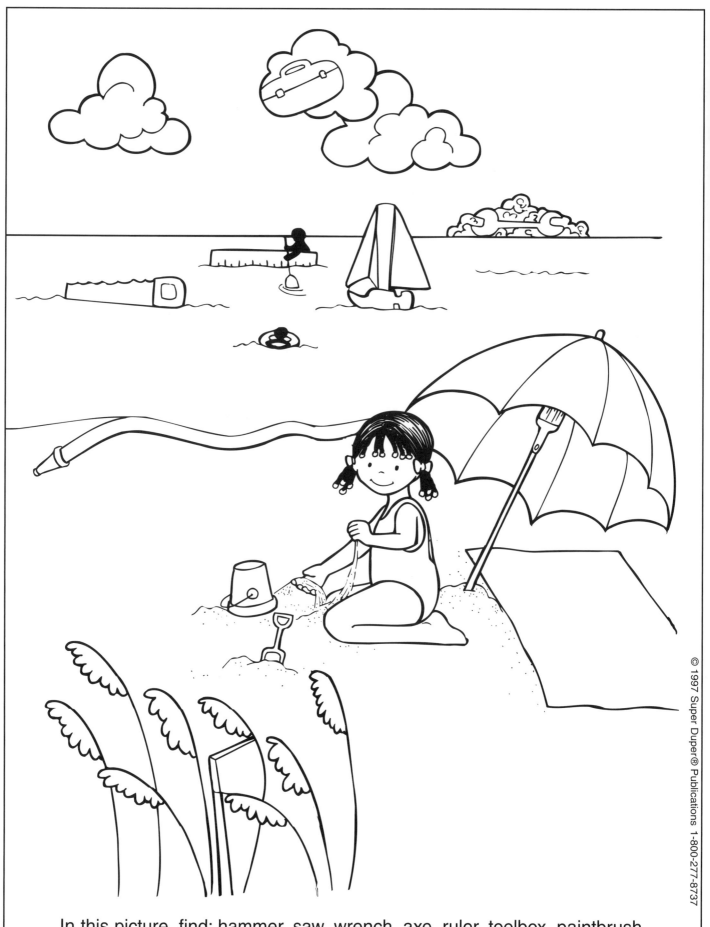

In this picture, find: hammer, saw, wrench, axe, ruler, toolbox, paintbrush, shovel, and garden hose.

114

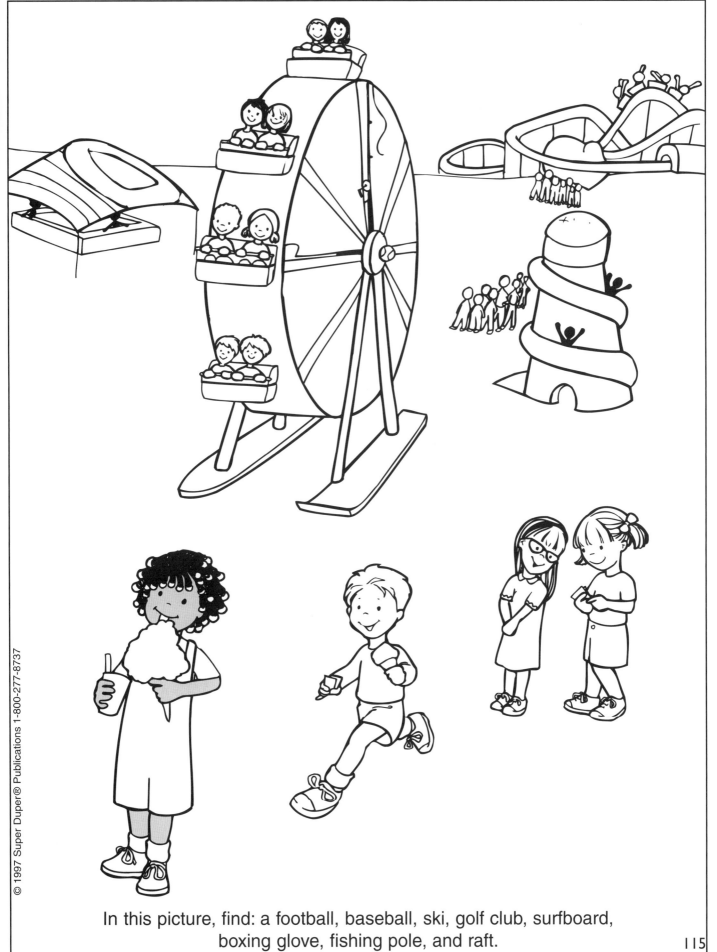

In this picture, find: a football, baseball, ski, golf club, surfboard, boxing glove, fishing pole, and raft.

115

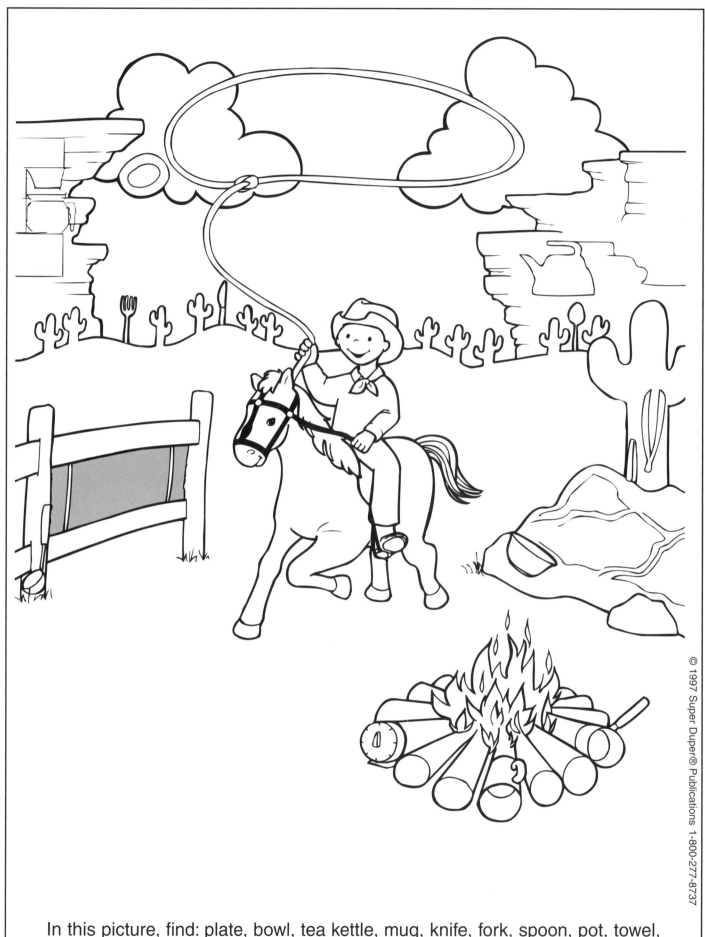

In this picture, find: plate, bowl, tea kettle, mug, knife, fork, spoon, pot, towel, coffee maker, chopsticks, ladle, tongs, and timer.

116

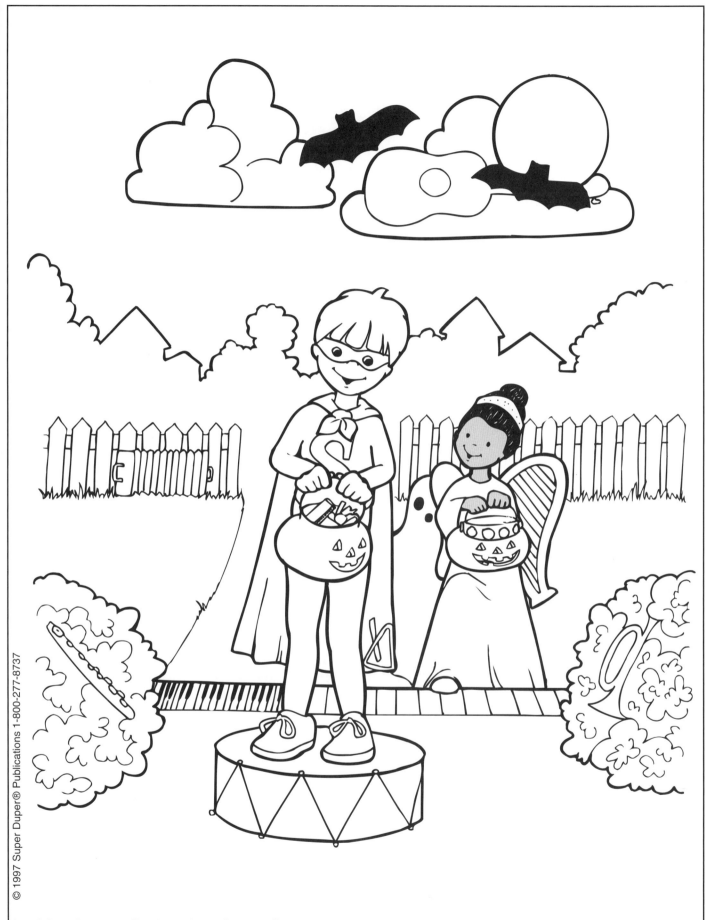

In this picture, find: guitar, harp, flute, drum, tambourine, trumpet, triangle, harmonica, keyboard, and accordion.

117

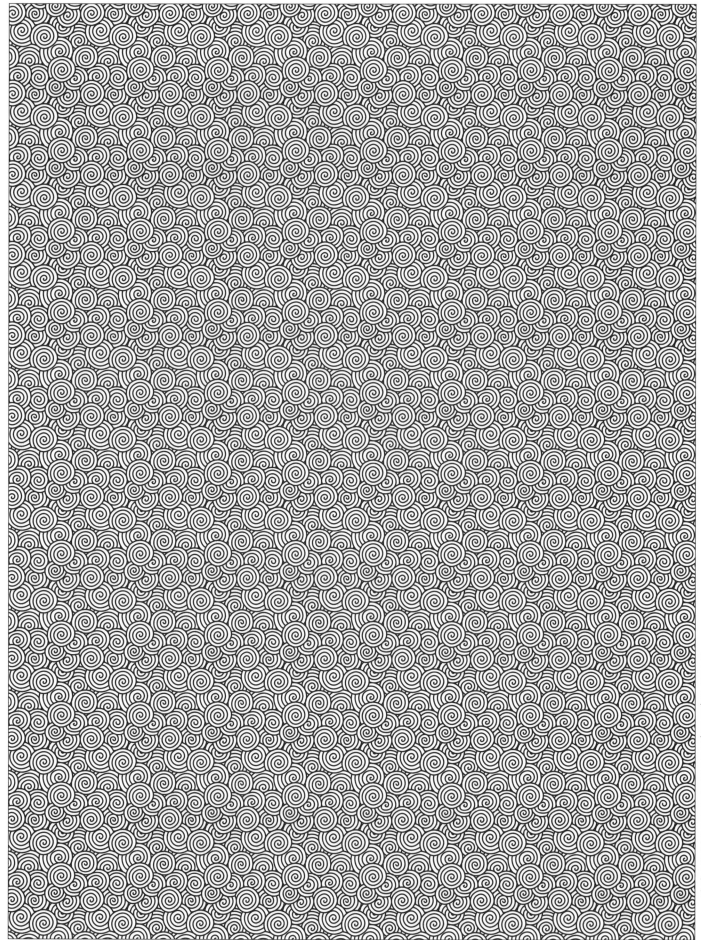

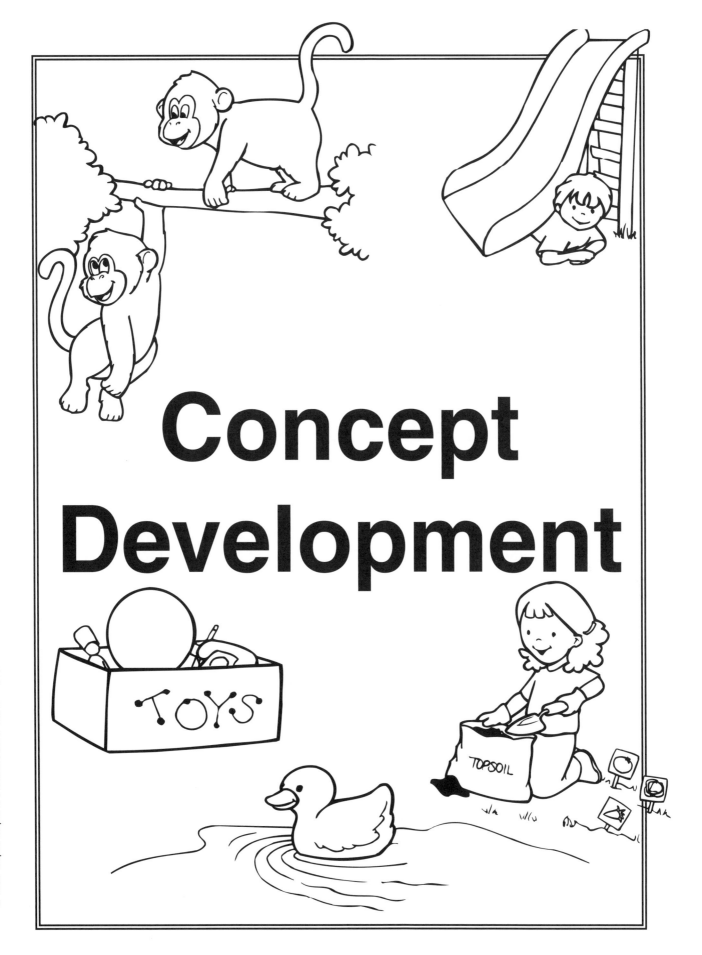

Concept Development

How To Use The Concept Section

1. Typically, a child is referred to the Speech-Language Pathologist, Special Education Teacher, or Bilingual/ ESL Specialist by a concerned individual. These individuals may be a parent, teacher, daycare provider, doctor, or relative who have noted the child's difficulty in producing words or sentences.

2. The specialist determines the child's language abilities through the use of various language assessments. Based on this evaluation, the specialist designs a specific remediation strategy to meet the individual needs of the child.

3. One of the more common techniques used by Speech-Language Pathologists is Auditory Bombardment. Many Speech-Language Pathologists have found this technique to be helpful with the remediation of both phonological and language delays. Using this section, the specialist selects the appropriate Auditory Bombardment sentence sheet for the child's therapy lesson. The illustrated blackline sentence page is then reproduced for teacher, student and parent use.

4. During the lesson, the specialist reads the selected Auditory Bombardment Sentences to the child. It is often helpful to present the sentences using a microphone/listening center arrangement with the child wearing an audio headset. The specialist reads the sentences through the microphone, with the volume slightly amplified. The common practice in a language lesson is to repeat the Auditory Bombardment activity twice – once at the beginning of the session and again as a final activity at the end of the session.

5. After the child has listened to the chosen Auditory Bombardment Sentences, the specialist may then want the child to produce the appropriate sentence structure. The specialist can use the included target concept pictures to elicit the appropriate verbalizations. Following a procedure similar to the one used in the vocabulary section, the specialist may wish to assemble the target concept pictures on a ring. (Please refer to the Vocabulary Section, page 2, for target concept picture assembly instructions.)

6. With each subsequent lesson, the specialist may wish to add additional target concept pictures to the ring.

7. To actively involve the parent in the remediation process, the specialist provides the parent with a copy of the day's Auditory Bombardment Sentences. Initially, the parent will receive a letter of explanation (Parent Letter) with child's first Auditory Bombardment Sentence Sheets. Coloring the pictures surrounding the bombardment sentences may serve as a positive reinforcement for the child.

8. The ringed target concept pictures can be sent home with the child for additional practice. The parents/guardians may be asked to return only the ringed target concept pictures for the next lesson.

9. Carry-over has been found to be an integral part of the remediation of language delays. With the use of this assessment-remediation-parent involvement loop, the specialist and the parent play a key role in the success of the child's remediation.

© 1997 Super Duper® Publications 1-800-277-8737

Dear Parents,

As a part of our speech therapy program, your child will be listening and producing various sentences. To encourage progress, you will be receiving sentence lists on a regular basis that are meant to be read to your child. The sentences in these lists have been carefully selected because they contain or emphasize a particular concept, such as "in." These lists, known as auditory bombardment lists, are to be read to your child in a slow and clear manner. Your child should not repeat these sentences but should quietly listen to them. It is suggested that you spend one to two minutes each day on this "read and listen" activity. One of the most important parts of this process is that you remember to praise your child for his/her good listening skills.

Each list is surrounded by pictures of the selected sentences. Allowing your child to color these pictures is a great reward for being a good listener! Please let me know if you have any questions. Thank you for your participation!

Sincerely,

Speech-Language Pathologist

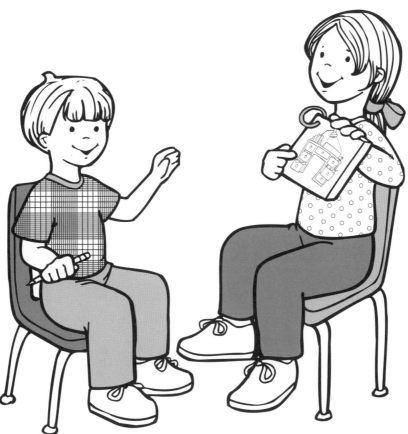

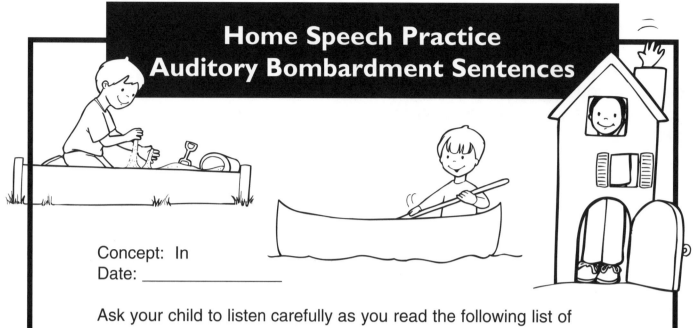

Home Speech Practice
Auditory Bombardment Sentences

Concept: In

Date: _____

Ask your child to listen carefully as you read the following list of sentences slowly and clearly. It is important that your child not repeat the sentences but just listen to them quietly. Please spend one to two minutes daily reading these sentences to your child. After listening to these sentences, your child may color the pictures on the page!

1. The boy is in the tree.
2. The boy is in the bed.
3. The boy is in the tent.
4. The boy is in the sandbox.
5. The boy is in the car.

6. The boy is in the bathtub.
7. The boy is in the swimming pool.
8. The boy is in the wheelchair.
9. The boy is in the canoe.
10. The boy is in the house.

Additional Comments/Helpful Hints:

_____

_____

_____

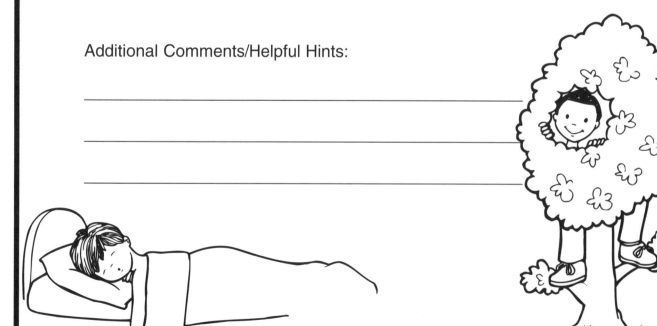

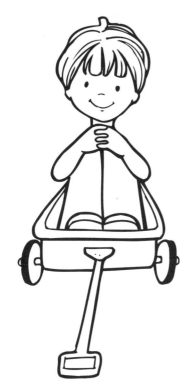

The boy is **in** the wagon.

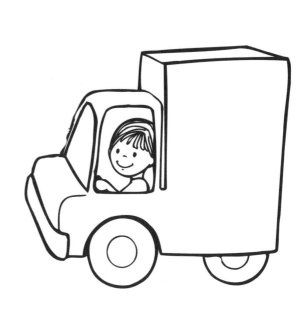

The boy is **in** the truck.

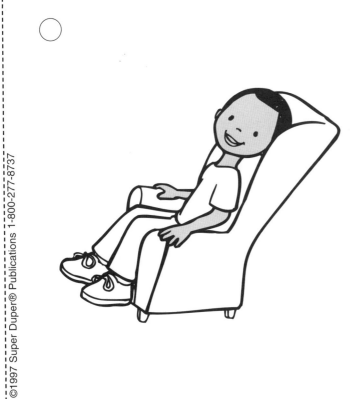

The boy is **in** the chair.

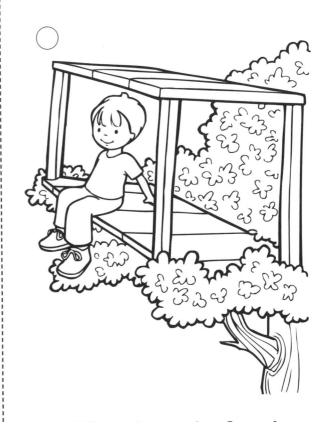

The boy is **in** the treehouse.

123

Home Speech Practice
Auditory Bombardment Sentences

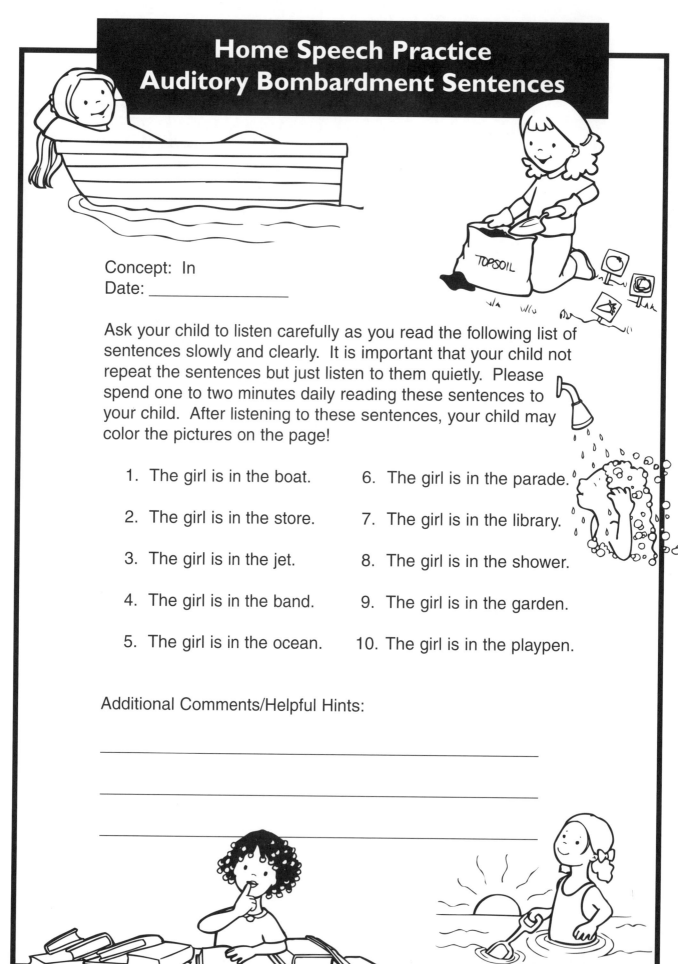

Concept: In

Date: _____

Ask your child to listen carefully as you read the following list of sentences slowly and clearly. It is important that your child not repeat the sentences but just listen to them quietly. Please spend one to two minutes daily reading these sentences to your child. After listening to these sentences, your child may color the pictures on the page!

1. The girl is in the boat.

2. The girl is in the store.

3. The girl is in the jet.

4. The girl is in the band.

5. The girl is in the ocean.

6. The girl is in the parade.

7. The girl is in the library.

8. The girl is in the shower.

9. The girl is in the garden.

10. The girl is in the playpen.

Additional Comments/Helpful Hints:

_____

_____

_____

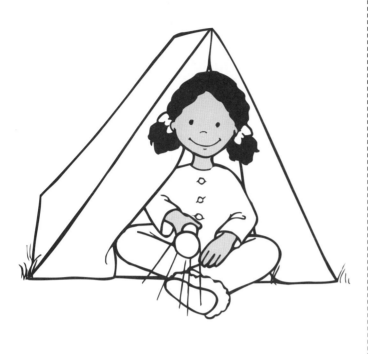

The girl is **in** the tent.

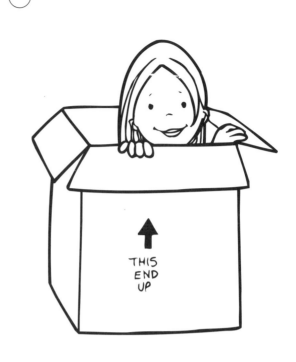

THIS
END
UP

The girl is **in** the box.

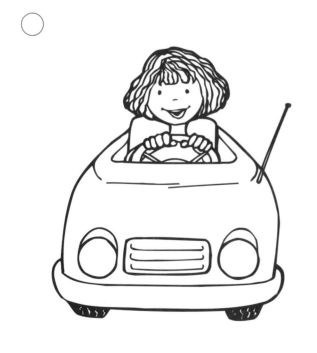

The girl is **in** the car.

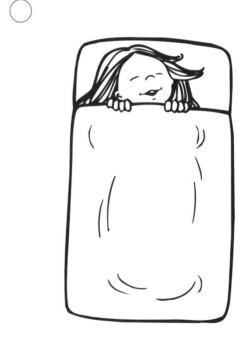

The girl is **in** the
sleeping bag.

125

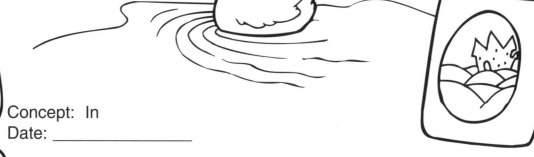

Home Speech Practice
Auditory Bombardment Sentences

Concept: In

Date: _____

Ask your child to listen carefully as you read the following list of sentences slowly and clearly. It is important that your child not repeat the sentences but just listen to them quietly. Please spend one to two minutes daily reading these sentences to your child. After listening to these sentences, your child may color the pictures on the page!

1. The ball is in the toy box.

2. The monkey is in the tree.

3. The duck is in the lake.

4. The shirt is in the drawer.

5. The picture is in the frame.

6. The pumpkin is in the window.

7. The flower is in the vase.

8. The car is in the garage.

9. The bear is in the cave.

10. The dog is in the doghouse.

Additional Comments/Helpful Hints:

_____

_____

_____

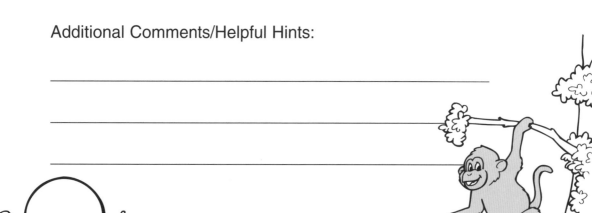

126

©1997 Super Duper® Publications 1-800-277-8737

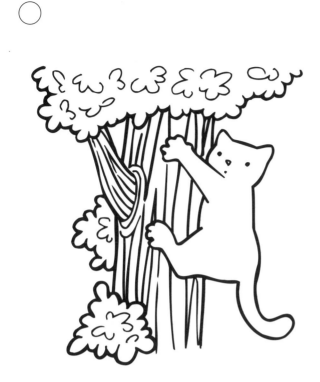

The cat is **in** the tree.

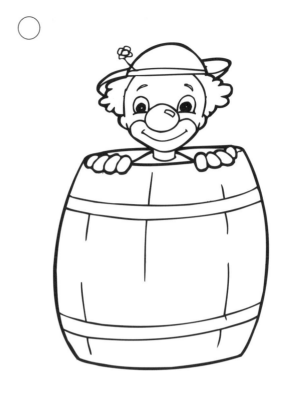

The clown is **in** the barrel.

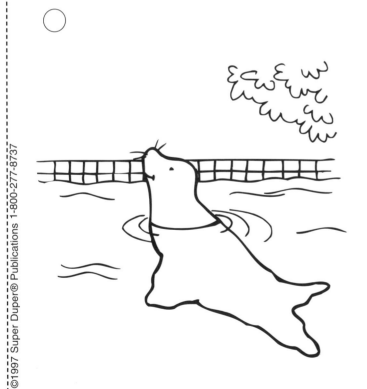

The seal is **in** the pool.

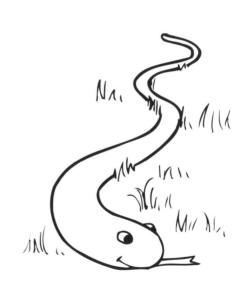

The snake is **in** the grass.

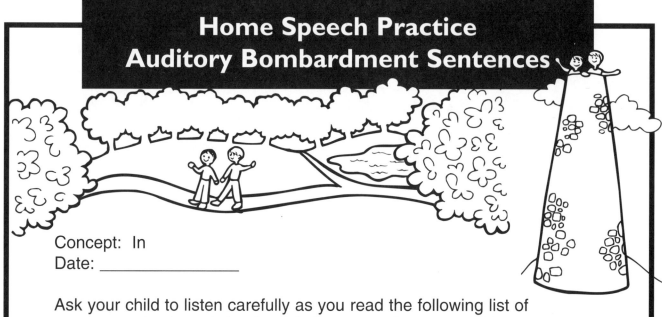

Home Speech Practice
Auditory Bombardment Sentences

Concept: In

Date: _____

Ask your child to listen carefully as you read the following list of sentences slowly and clearly. It is important that your child not repeat the sentences but just listen to them quietly. Please spend one to two minutes daily reading these sentences to your child. After listening to these sentences, your child may color the pictures on the page!

1. The boys are in the parade.
2. The boys are in the park.
3. The boys are in the garage.
4. The boys are in the sailboat.
5. The boys are in the tent.
6. The boys are in the shade.
7. The boys are in the cafeteria.
8. The boys are in the mountains.
9. The boys are in the tower.
10. The boys are in the office.

Additional Comments/Helpful Hints:

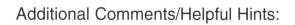

_____

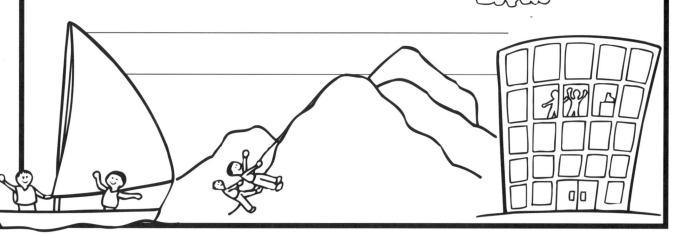

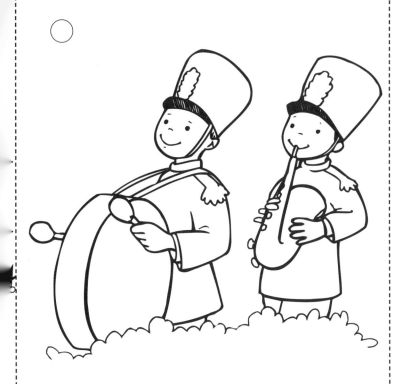

The boys are **in** the band.

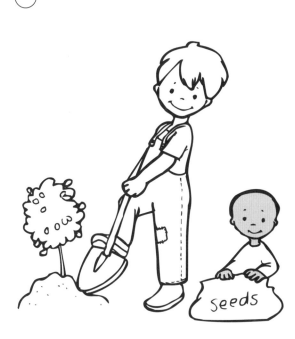

The boys are **in** the garden.

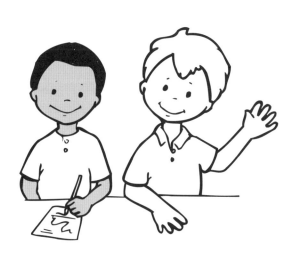

The boys are **in** the classroom.

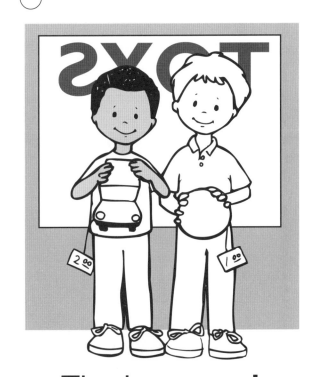

The boys are **in** the toy store.

129

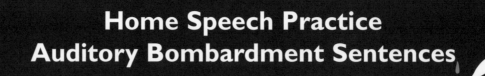

Home Speech Practice
Auditory Bombardment Sentences

Concept: In

Date: _____

Ask your child to listen carefully as you read the following list of sentences slowly and clearly. It is important that your child not repeat the sentences but just listen to them quietly. Please spend one to two minutes daily reading these sentences to your child. After listening to these sentences, your child may color the pictures on the page!

1. The girls are in the snow.
2. The girls are in the cave.
3. The girls are in the forest.
4. The girls are in the rain.
5. The girls are in the school.
6. The girls are in the taxi.
7. The girls are in the choir.
8. The girls are in the attic.
9. The girls are in the circus.
10. The girls are in the barn.

Additional Comments/Helpful Hints:

_____

_____

_____

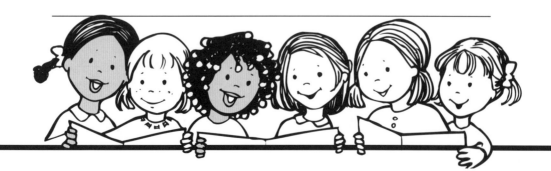

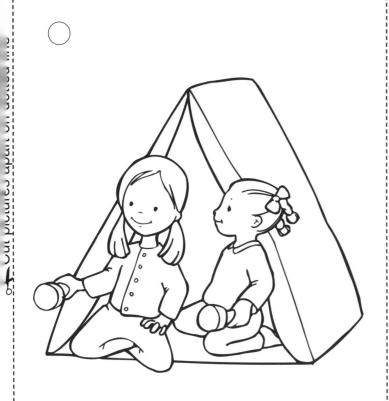

The girls are **in** the tent.

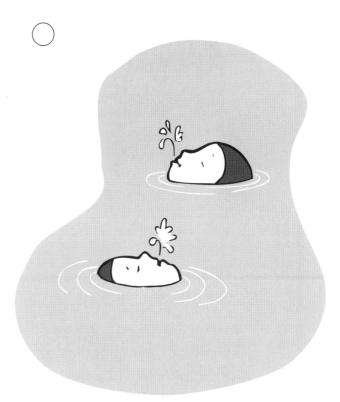

The girls are **in** the pool.

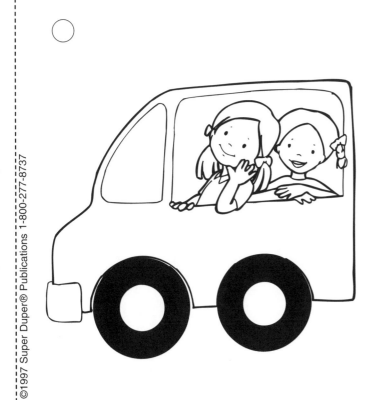

The girls are **in** the van.

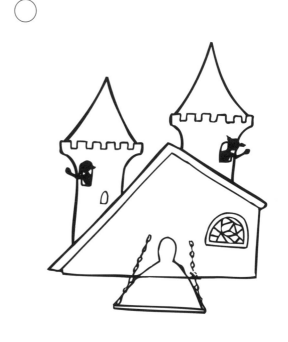

The girls are **in** the castle.

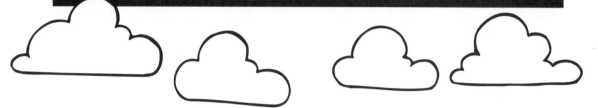

Home Speech Practice
Auditory Bombardment Sentences

Concept: In

Date: _____

Ask your child to listen carefully as you read the following list of sentences slowly and clearly. It is important that your child not repeat the sentences but just listen to them quietly. Please spend one to two minutes daily reading these sentences to your child. After listening to these sentences, your child may color the pictures on the page!

1. The ducks are in the pond.   6. The birds are in the tree.

2. The horses are in the barn.   7. The letters are in the mailbox.

3. The pies are in the oven.   8. The clouds are in the sky.

4. The donuts are in the box.   9. The books are in the desk.

5. The camels are in the desert. 10. The costumes are in the closet.

Additional Comments/Helpful Hints:

_____

_____

_____

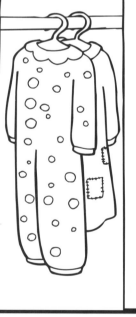

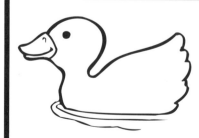

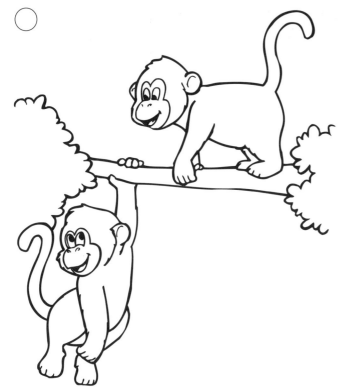

The monkeys are **in** the tree.

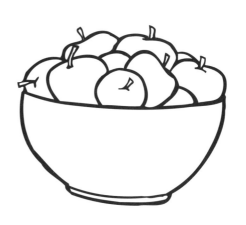

The apples are **in** the bowl.

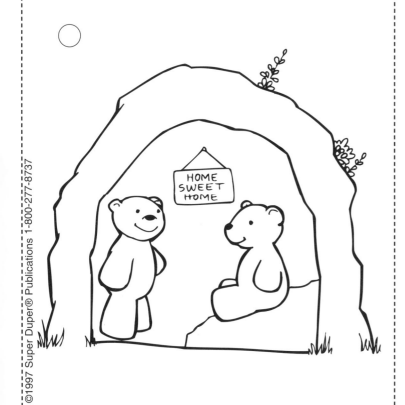

The bears are **in** the cave.

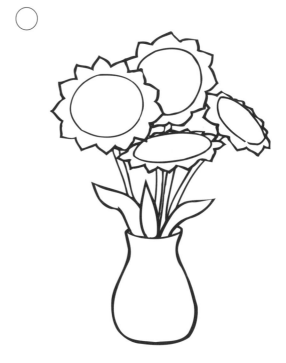

The flowers are **in** the vase.

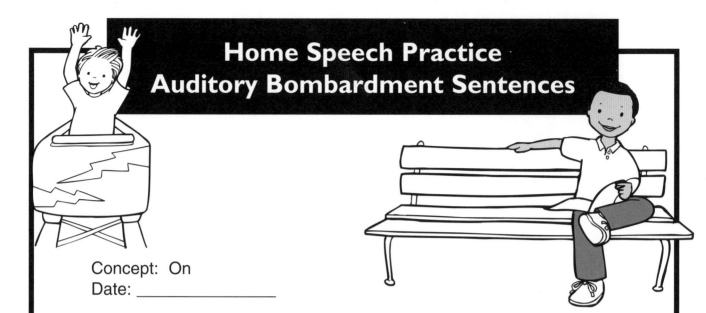

Home Speech Practice
Auditory Bombardment Sentences

Concept: On

Date: _____

Ask your child to listen carefully as you read the following list of sentences slowly and clearly. It is important that your child not repeat the sentences but just listen to them quietly. Please spend one to two minutes daily reading these sentences to your child. After listening to these sentences, your child may color the pictures on the page!

1. The boy is on the bench.
2. The boy is on the floor.
3. The boy is on the swing.
4. The boy is on the roof.
5. The boy is on the phone.
6. The boy is on the playground.
7. The boy is on the diving board.
8. The boy is on the skateboard.
9. The boy is on the roller coaster.
10. The boy is on the grass.

Additional Comments/Helpful Hints:

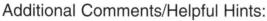

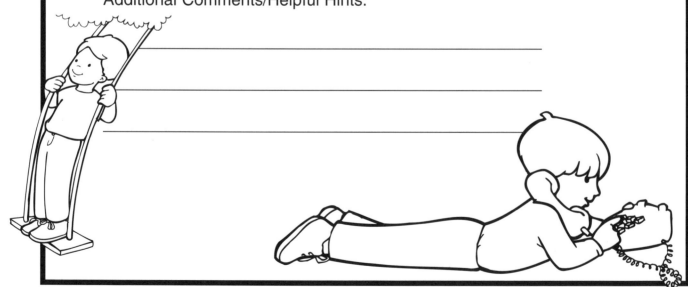

134

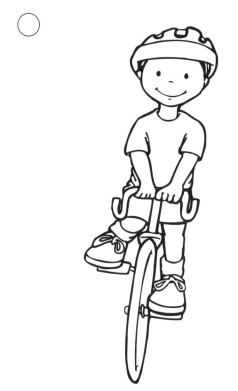

The boy is **on** the couch.

The boy is **on** the bike.

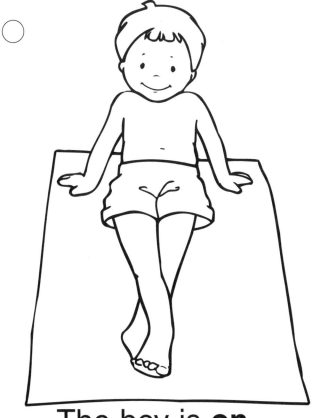

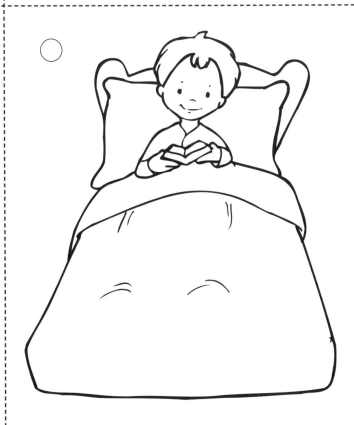

The boy is **on** the towel.

The boy is **on** the bed.

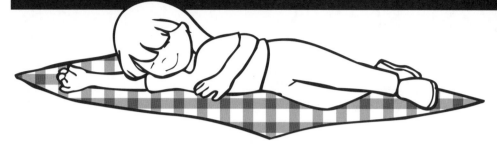

Concept: On

Date: _____

Ask your child to listen carefully as you read the following list of sentences slowly and clearly. It is important that your child not repeat the sentences but just listen to them quietly. Please spend one to two minutes daily reading these sentences to your child. After listening to these sentences, your child may color the pictures on the page!

1. The girl is on the chair.

2. The girl is on the tractor.

3. The girl is on the scooter.

4. The girl is on the trampoline.

5. The girl is on the stairs.

6. The girl is on the scale.

7. The girl is on the stage.

8. The girl is on the ladder.

9. The girl is on the blanket.

10. The girl is on the fence.

Additional Comments/Helpful Hints:

_____

_____

_____

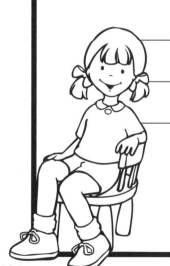

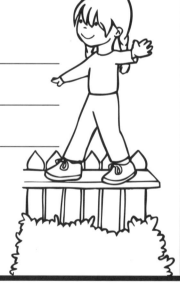

©1997 Super Duper® Publications 1-800-277-8737

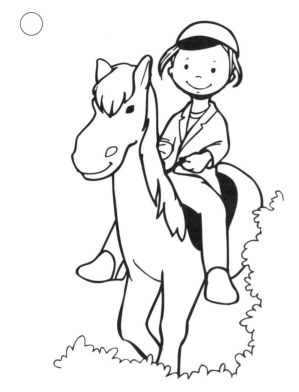

The girl is **on** the horse.

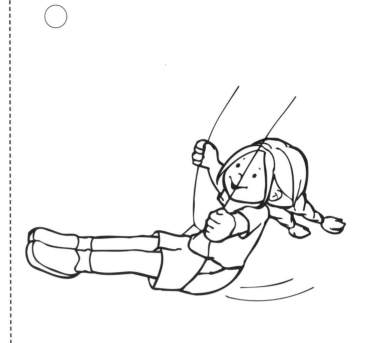

The girl is **on** the swing.

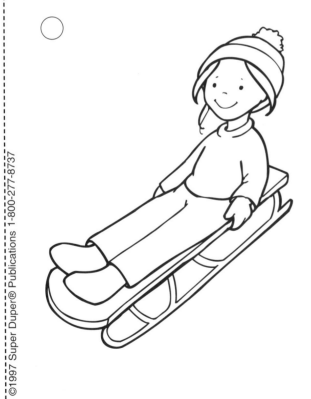

The girl is **on** the sled.

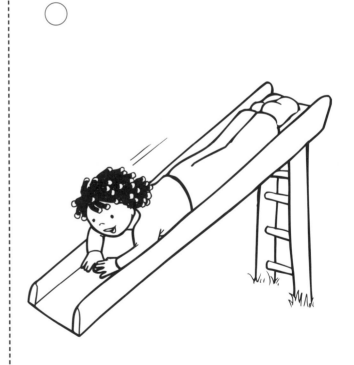

The girl is **on** the slide.

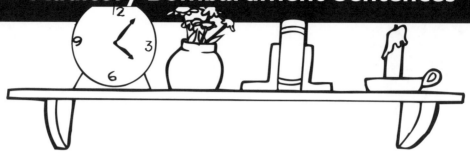

Home Speech Practice
Auditory Bombardment Sentences

Concept: On

Date: _____

Ask your child to listen carefully as you read the following list of sentences slowly and clearly. It is important that your child not repeat the sentences but just listen to them quietly. Please spend one to two minutes daily reading these sentences to your child. After listening to these sentences, your child may color the pictures on the page!

1. The butterfly is on the flower.
2. The bird is on the branch.
3. The coat is on the hanger.
4. The book is on the shelf.
5. The pumpkin is on the porch.
6. The airplane is on the runway.
7. The pillow is on the bed.
8. The computer is on the desk.
9. The cat is on the couch.
10. The truck is on the road.

Additional Comments/Helpful Hints:

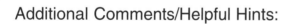

_____

_____

_____

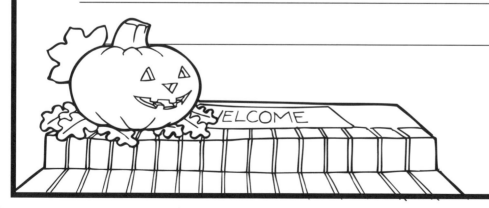

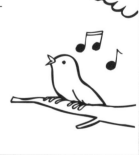

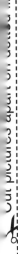

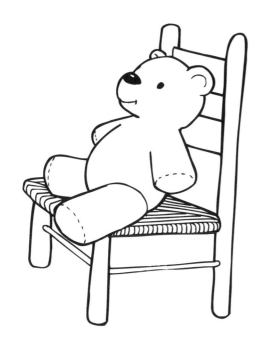

The teddy bear is **on** the chair.

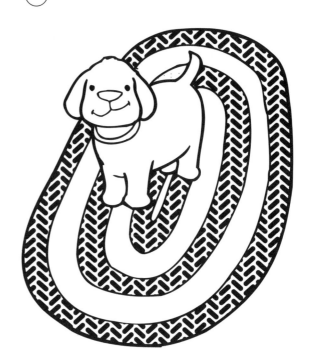

The dog is **on** the rug.

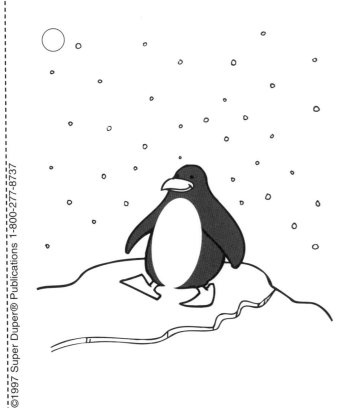

The penguin is **on** the ice.

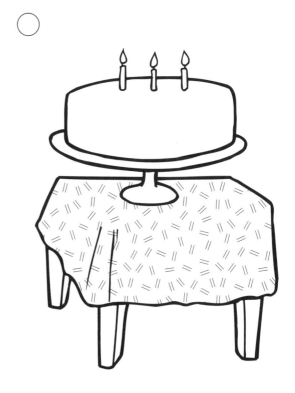

The cake is **on** the table.

139

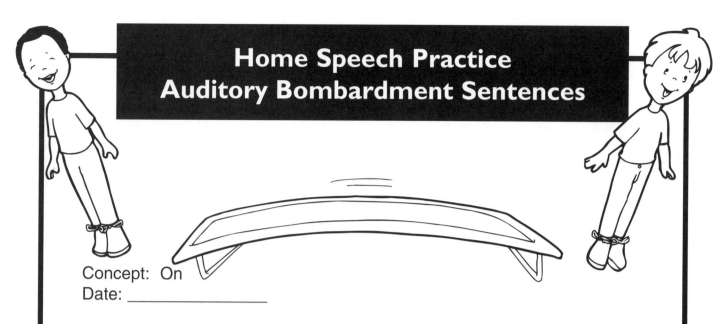

Home Speech Practice
Auditory Bombardment Sentences

Concept: On

Date: _____

Ask your child to listen carefully as you read the following list of sentences slowly and clearly. It is important that your child not repeat the sentences but just listen to them quietly. Please spend one to two minutes daily reading these sentences to your child. After listening to these sentences, your child may color the pictures on the page!

1. The boys are on the slide.

2. The boys are on the horse.

3. The boys are on the seesaw.

4. The boys are on the motorcycle.

5. The boys are on the bridge.

6. The boys are on the trampoline.

7. The boys are on the field.

8. The boys are on the towel.

9. The boys are on the bus.

10. The boys are on the Ferris wheel.

Additional Comments/Helpful Hints:

_____

_____

_____

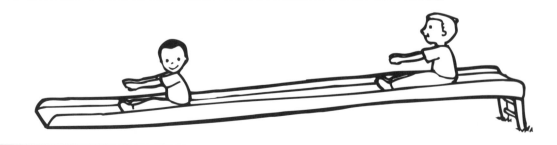

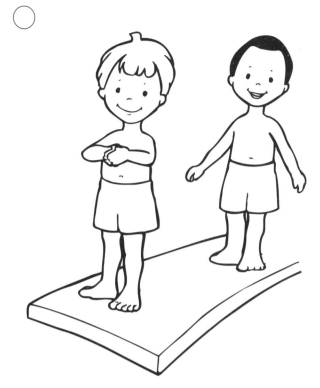

The boys are **on** the diving board.

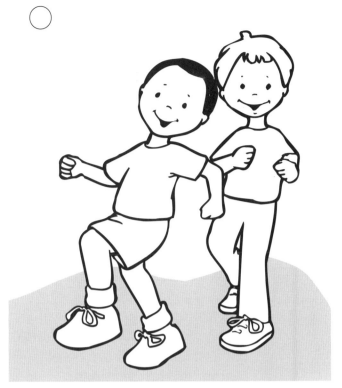

The boys are **on** the playground.

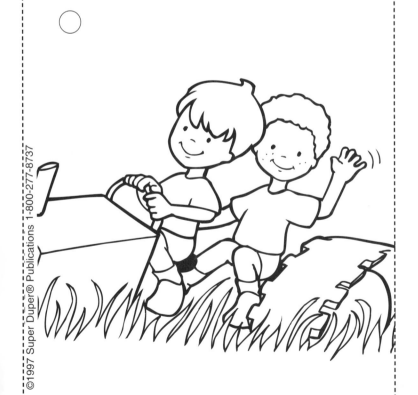

The boys are **on** the tractor.

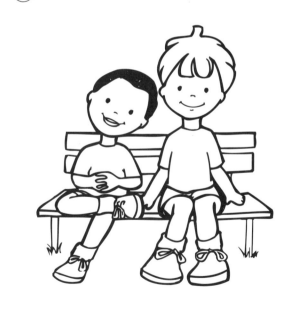

The boys are **on** the bench.

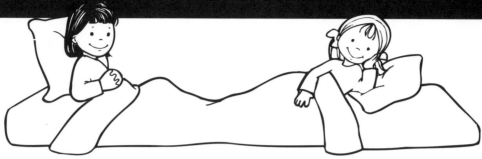

Home Speech Practice
Auditory Bombardment Sentences

Concept: On

Date: _____

Ask your child to listen carefully as you read the following list of sentences slowly and clearly. It is important that your child not repeat the sentences but just listen to them quietly. Please spend one to two minutes daily reading these sentences to your child. After listening to these sentences, your child may color the pictures on the page!

1. The girls are on the couch.
2. The girls are on the sailboat.
3. The girls are on the bed.
4. The girls are on the sled.
5. The girls are on the hill.

6. The girls are on the roller coaster.
7. The girls are on the porch.
8. The girls are on the beach.
9. The girls are on the carpet.
10. The girls are on the team.

Additional Comments/Helpful Hints:

_____

_____

_____

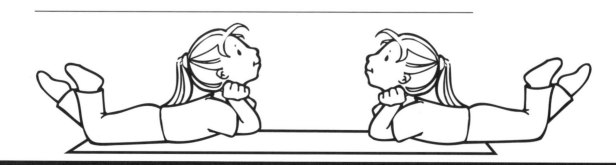

©1997 Super Duper® Publications 1-800-277-8737

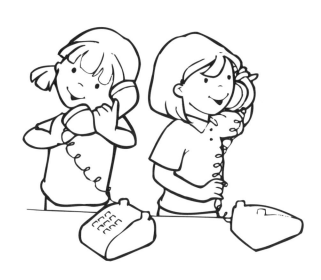

The girls are **on** the phone.

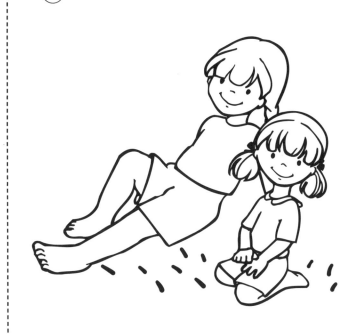

The girls are **on** the grass.

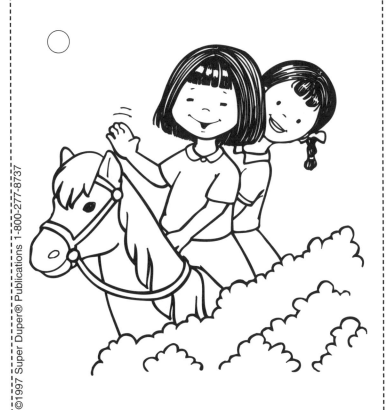

The girls are **on** the horse.

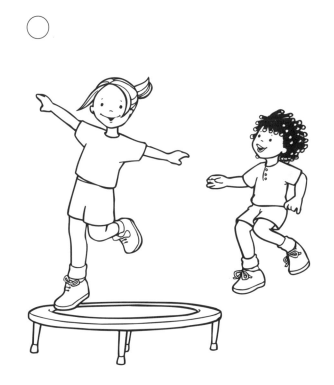

The girls are **on** the trampoline.

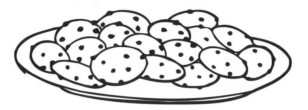

Home Speech Practice
Auditory Bombardment Sentences

Concept: On

Date: _____

Ask your child to listen carefully as you read the following list of sentences slowly and clearly. It is important that your child not repeat the sentences but just listen to them quietly. Please spend one to two minutes daily reading these sentences to your child. After listening to these sentences, your child may color the pictures on the page!

1. The napkins are on the table.
2. The ladybugs are on the leaf.
3. The pictures are on the wall.
4. The cookies are on the plate.
5. The trophies are on the shelf.
6. The rabbits are on the grass.
7. The pencils are on the desk.
8. The magnets are on the refrigerator.
9. The shells are on the beach.
10. The keys are on the chain.

Additional Comments/Helpful Hints:

_____

_____

_____

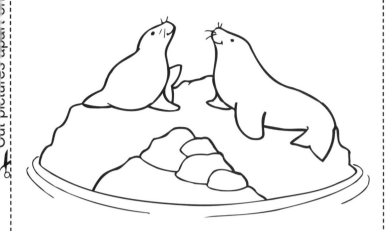

The seals are **on** the rock.

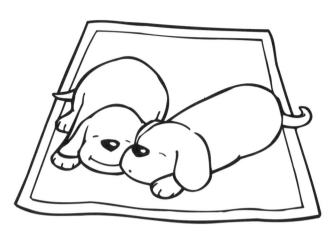

The dogs are **on** the blanket.

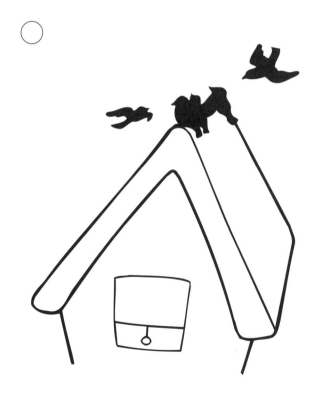

The birds are **on** the roof.

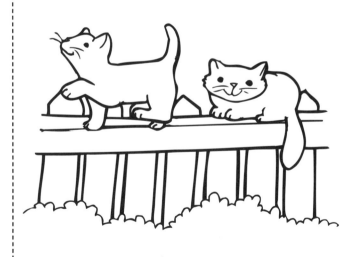

The cats are **on** the fence.

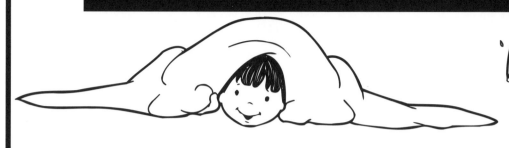

Home Speech Practice
Auditory Bombardment Sentences

Concept: Under

Date: _____

Ask your child to listen carefully as you read the following list of sentences slowly and clearly. It is important that your child not repeat the sentences but just listen to them quietly. Please spend one to two minutes daily reading these sentences to your child. After listening to these sentences, your child may color the pictures on the page!

1. The boy is under the bridge.
2. The boy is under the desk.
3. The boy is under the chair.
4. The boy is under the sign.
5. The boy is under the table.
6. The boy is under the blanket.
7. The boy is under the balcony.
8. The boy is under the umbrella.
9. The boy is under the stairs.
10. The boy is under the couch.

Additional Comments/Helpful Hints:

_____

_____

_____

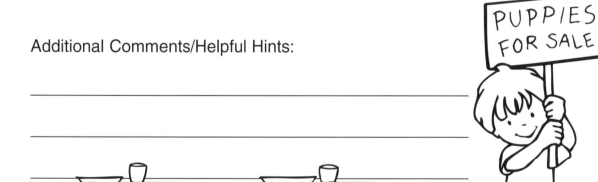

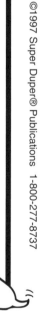

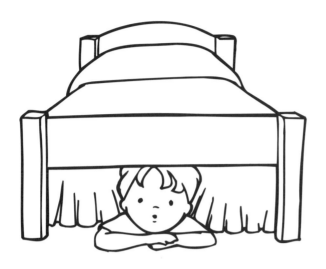

The boy is **under** the bed.

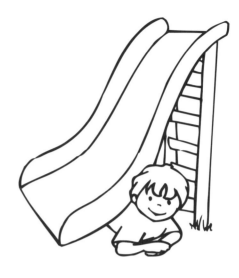

The boy is **under** the slide.

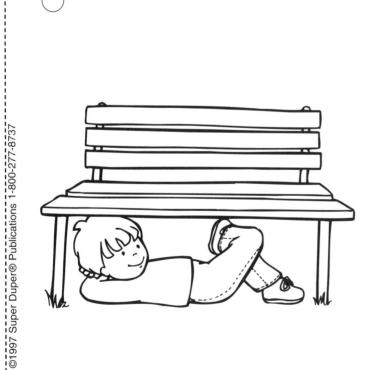

The boy is **under** the bench.

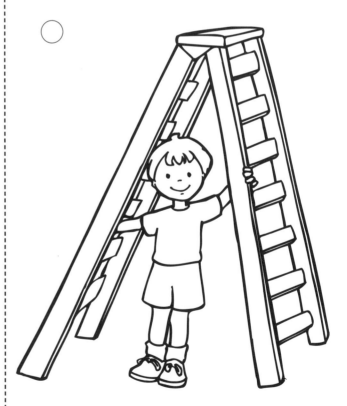

The boy is **under** the ladder.

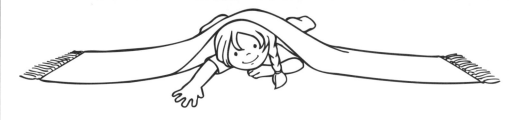

Home Speech Practice
Auditory Bombardment Sentences

Concept: Under

Date: _____

Ask your child to listen carefully as you read the following list of sentences slowly and clearly. It is important that your child not repeat the sentences but just listen to them quietly. Please spend one to two minutes daily reading these sentences to your child. After listening to these sentences, your child may color the pictures on the page!

1. The girl is under the rug.   6. The girl is under the sink.

2. The girl is under the water.   7. The girl is under the flag.

3. The girl is under the bench.   8. The girl is under the sign.

4. The girl is under the lights.   9. The girl is under the kite.

5. The girl is under the fan.   10. The girl is under the balloon.

Additional Comments/Helpful Hints:

_____

_____

_____

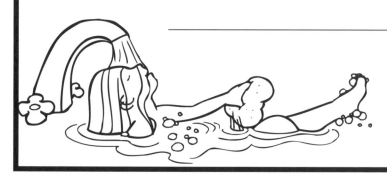

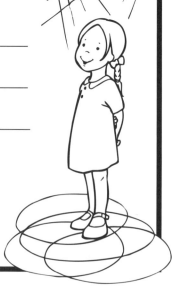

©1997 Super Duper® Publications 1-800-277-8737

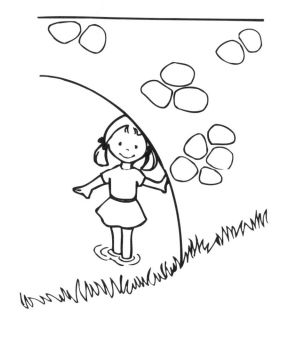

The girl is **under** the bridge.

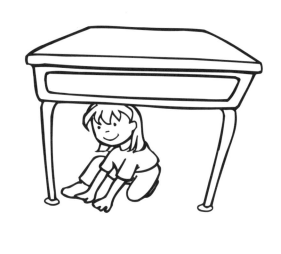

The girl is **under** the desk.

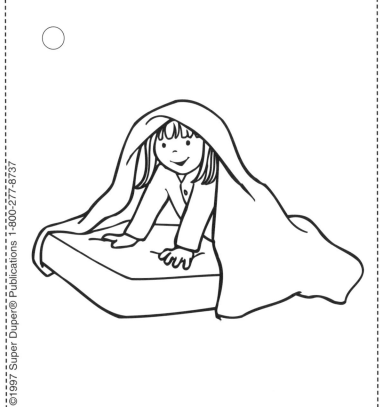

The girl is **under** the sheet.

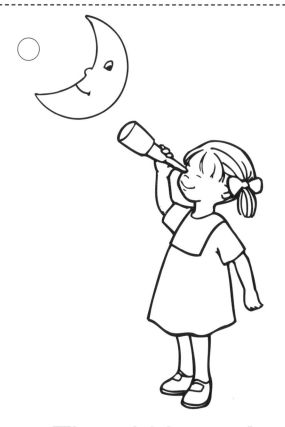

The girl is **under** the moon.

Home Speech Practice
Auditory Bombardment Sentences

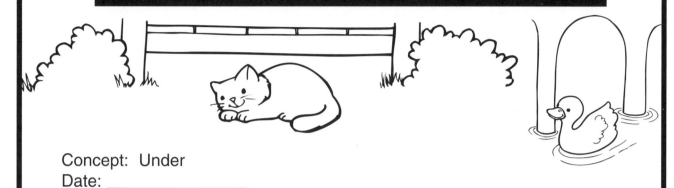

Concept: Under

Date: _____

Ask your child to listen carefully as you read the following list of sentences slowly and clearly. It is important that your child not repeat the sentences but just listen to them quietly. Please spend one to two minutes daily reading these sentences to your child. After listening to these sentences, your child may color the pictures on the page!

1. The dog is under the stool.
2. The key is under the mat.
3. The napkin is under the fork.
4. The saucer is under the cup.
5. The cat is under the porch.
6. The mouse is under the box.
7. The ball is under the bush.
8. The newspaper is under the bench.
9. The tooth is under the pillow.
10. The duck is under the bridge.

Additional Comments/Helpful Hints:

_____

_____

_____

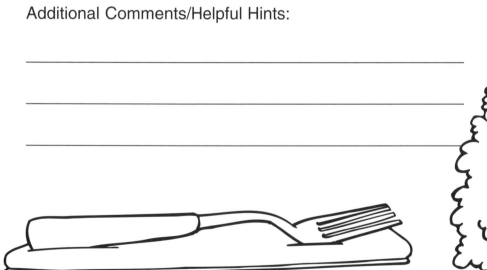

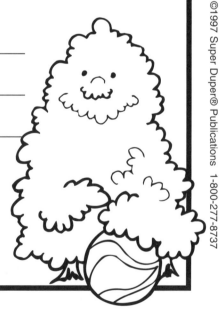

150

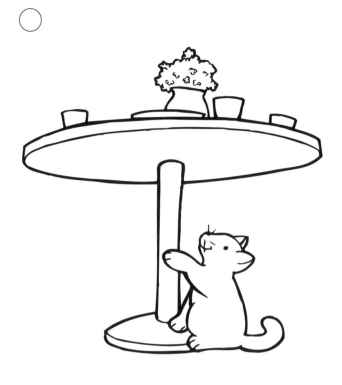

The kitten is **under** the table.

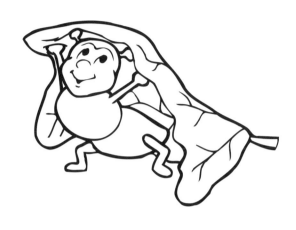

The ant is **under** the leaf.

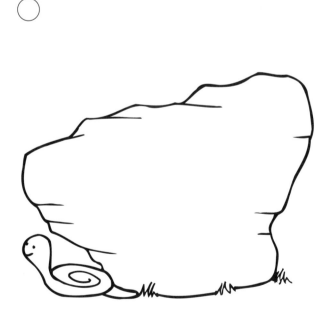

The snake is **under** the rock.

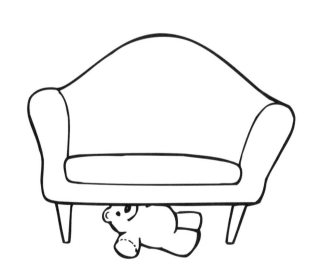

The teddy bear is **under** the couch. 151

Home Speech Practice
Auditory Bombardment Sentences

Concept: Under

Date: _____

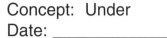

Ask your child to listen carefully as you read the following list of sentences slowly and clearly. It is important that your child not repeat the sentences but just listen to them quietly. Please spend one to two minutes daily reading these sentences to your child. After listening to these sentences, your child may color the pictures on the page!

1. The boys are under the slide.

2. The boys are under the balcony.

3. The boys are under the counter.

4. The boys are under the roof.

5. The boys are under the parachute.

6. The boys are under the table.

7. The boys are under the bed.

8. The boys are under the fan.

9. The boys are under the arch.

10. The boys are under the stars.

Additional Comments/Helpful Hints:

_____

_____

_____

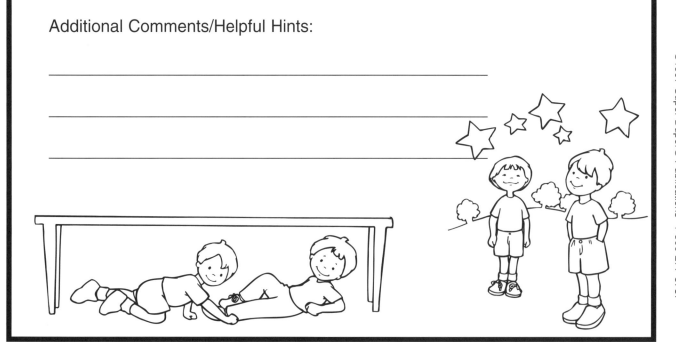

©1997 Super Duper® Publications 1-800-277-8737

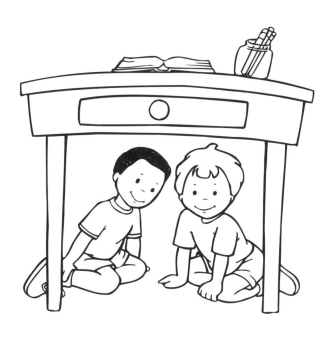

The boys are **under** the desk.

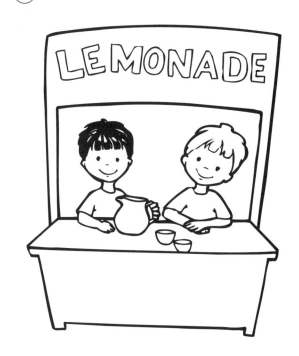

The boys are **under** the sign.

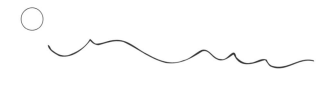
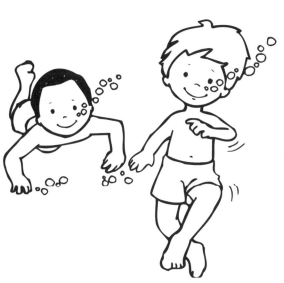

The boys are **under** the water.

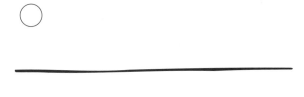
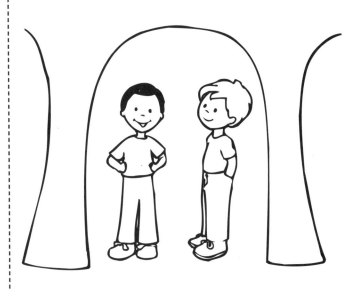

The boys are **under** the bridge.

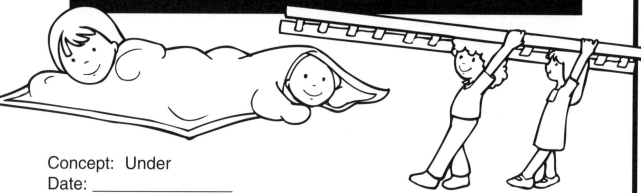

Home Speech Practice
Auditory Bombardment Sentences

Concept: Under

Date: _____

Ask your child to listen carefully as you read the following list of sentences slowly and clearly. It is important that your child not repeat the sentences but just listen to them quietly. Please spend one to two minutes daily reading these sentences to your child. After listening to these sentences, your child may color the pictures on the page!

1. The girls are under the ladder.
2. The girls are under the box.
3. The girls are under the picture.
4. The girls are under the balcony.
5. The girls are under the slide.
6. The girls are under the stars.
7. The girls are under the desk.
8. The girls are under the bridge.
9. The girls are under the bench.
10. The girls are under the blanket.

Additional Comments/Helpful Hints:

_____

_____

_____

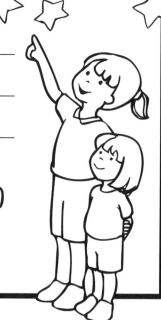

154

©1997 Super Duper® Publications 1-800-277-8737

©1997 Super Duper® Publications 1-800-277-8737

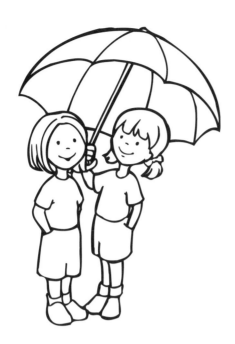

The girls are **under** the umbrella.

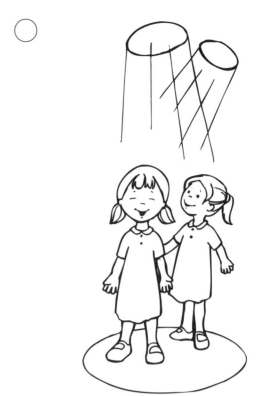

The girls are **under** the lights.

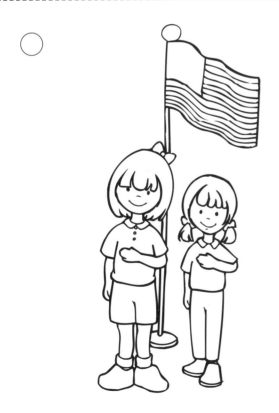

The girls are **under** the flag.

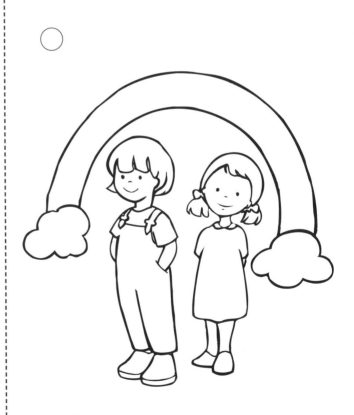

The girls are **under** the rainbow.

155

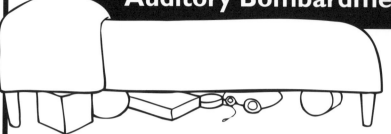

Home Speech Practice
Auditory Bombardment Sentences

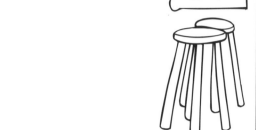

Concept: Under

Date: _____

Ask your child to listen carefully as you read the following list of sentences slowly and clearly. It is important that your child not repeat the sentences but just listen to them quietly. Please spend one to two minutes daily reading these sentences to your child. After listening to these sentences, your child may color the pictures on the page!

1. The cats are under the porch.

2. The napkins are under the plate.

3. The keys are under the rug.

4. The worms are under the ground.

5. The toys are under the bed.

6. The birds are under the bench.

7. The stools are under the counter.

8. The books are under the desk.

9. The frogs are under the bush.

10. The stuffed animals are under the blanket.

Additional Comments/Helpful Hints:

_____

_____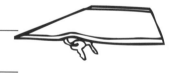

_____

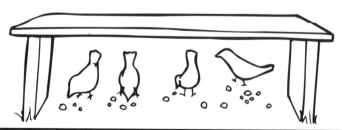

©1997 Super Duper® Publications 1-800-277-8737

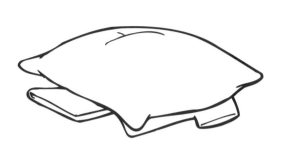

The pajamas are **under** the pillow.

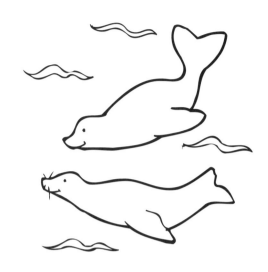

The seals are **under** the water.

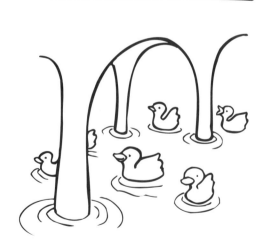

The ducks are **under** the bridge.

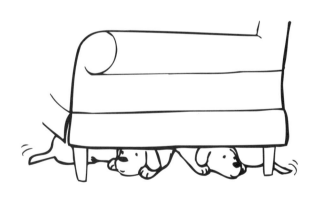

The dogs are **under** the couch.

©1997 Super Duper® Publications 1-800-277-8737

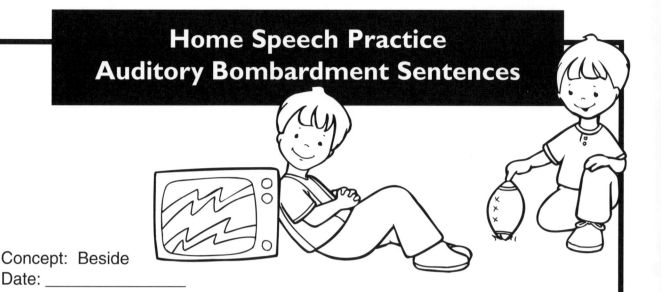

Home Speech Practice
Auditory Bombardment Sentences

Concept: Beside
Date: _____

Ask your child to listen carefully as you read the following list of sentences slowly and clearly. It is important that your child not repeat the sentences but just listen to them quietly. Please spend one to two minutes daily reading these sentences to your child. After listening to these sentences, your child may color the pictures on the page!

1. The boy is beside the bicycle

2. The boy is beside the dog.

3. The boy is beside the slide.

4. The boy is beside the television.

5. The boy is beside the ladder.

6. The boy is beside the ball.

7. The boy is beside the house.

8. The boy is beside the stool.

9. The boy is beside the bookshelf.

10. The boy is beside the basketball hoop.

Additional Comments/Helpful Hints:

_____

_____

_____

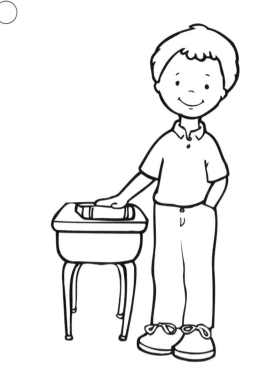

The boy is **beside** the desk.

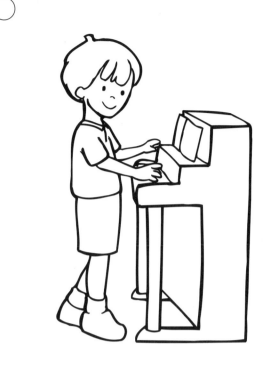

The boy is **beside** the piano.

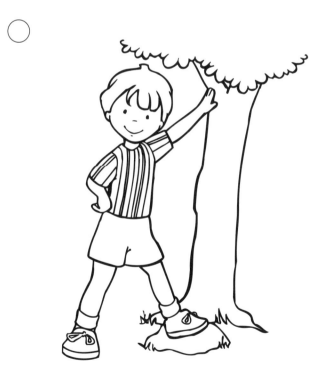

The boy is **beside** the tree.

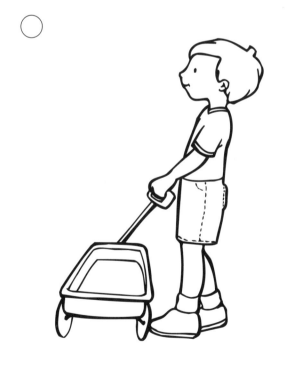

The boy is **beside** the wagon.

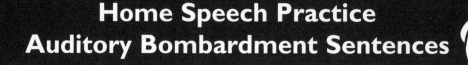

Home Speech Practice
Auditory Bombardment Sentences

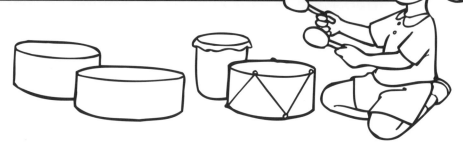

Concept: Beside

Date: _____

Ask your child to listen carefully as you read the following list of sentences slowly and clearly. It is important that your child not repeat the sentences but just listen to them quietly. Please spend one to two minutes daily reading these sentences to your child. After listening to these sentences, your child may color the pictures on the page!

1. The girl is beside the scooter.
2. The girl is beside the flower.
3. The girl is beside the horse.
4. The girl is beside the stage.
5. The girl is beside the train.
6. The girl is beside the statue.
7. The girl is beside the clown.
8. The girl is beside the pool.
9. The girl is beside the drums.
10. The girl is beside the mailbox.

Additional Comments/Helpful Hints:

_____

_____

_____

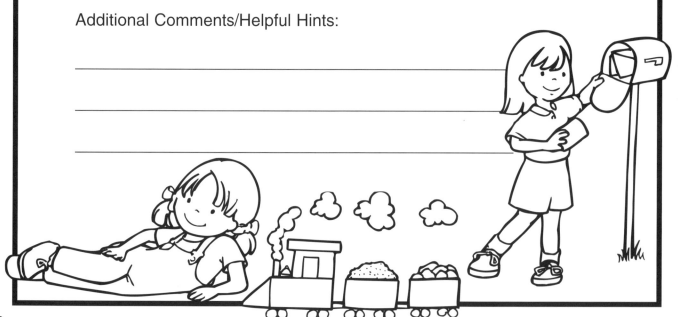

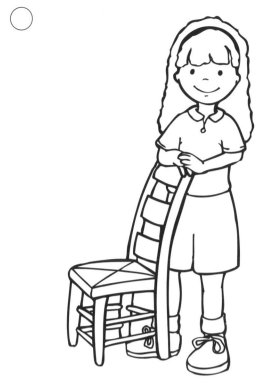

The girl is **beside** the chair.

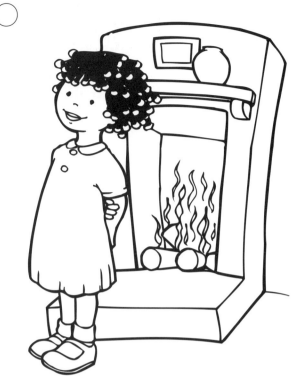

The girl is **beside** the fireplace.

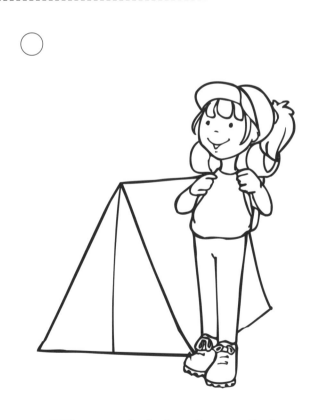

The girl is **beside** the tent.

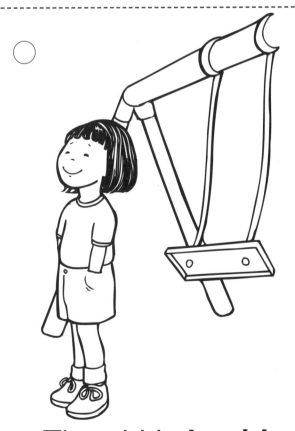

The girl is **beside** the swing.

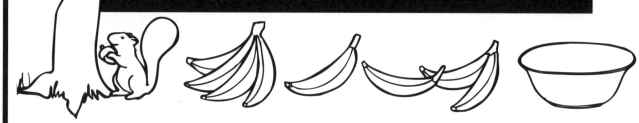

Concept: Beside

Date: _____

Ask your child to listen carefully as you read the following list of sentences slowly and clearly. It is important that your child not repeat the sentences but just listen to them quietly. Please spend one to two minutes daily reading these sentences to your child. After listening to these sentences, your child may color the pictures on the page!

1. The squirrel is beside the tree.

2. The car is beside the truck.

3. The skunk is beside the bush.

4. The book is beside the backpack.

5. The bananas are beside the bowl.

6. The flower is beside the house.

7. The seal is beside the rock.

8. The cat is beside the pumpkin.

9. The motorcycle is beside the garage.

10. The lamp is beside the chair.

Additional Comments/Helpful Hints:

_____

_____

_____

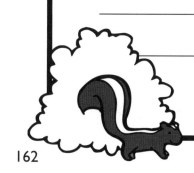

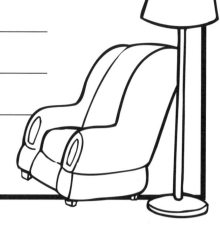

162

©1997 Super Duper® Publications 1-800-277-8737

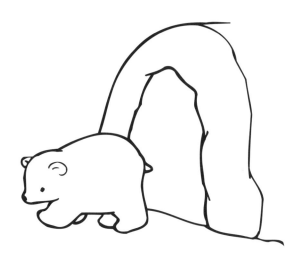

The bear is **beside** the cave.

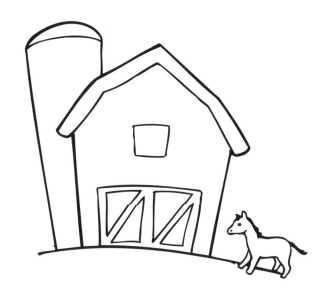

The horse is **beside** the barn.

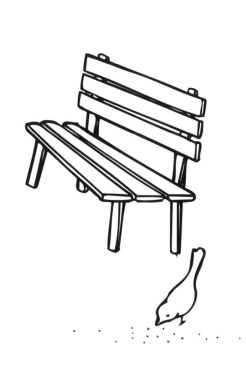

The bird is **beside** the bench.

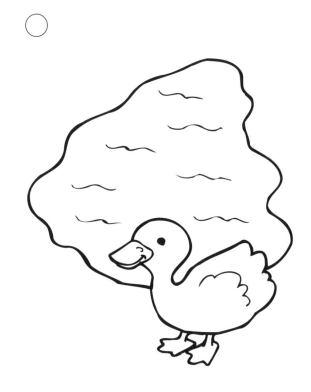

The duck is **beside** the pond.

163

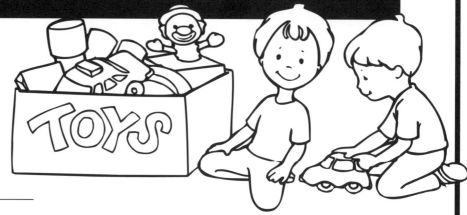

Home Speech Practice
Auditory Bombardment Sentences

Concept: Beside
Date: _____

Ask your child to listen carefully as you read the following list of sentences slowly and clearly. It is important that your child not repeat the sentences but just listen to them quietly. Please spend one to two minutes daily reading these sentences to your child. After listening to these sentences, your child may color the pictures on the page!

1. The boys are beside the bus.
2. The boys are beside the sign.
3. The boys are beside the clock.
4. The boys are beside the tractor.
5. The boys are beside the flag.
6. The boys are beside the door.
7. The boys are beside the bed.
8. The boys are beside the toy box.
9. The boys are beside the couch.
10. The boys are beside the aquarium.

Additional Comments/Helpful Hints:

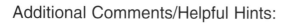

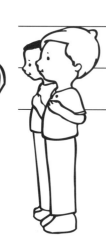

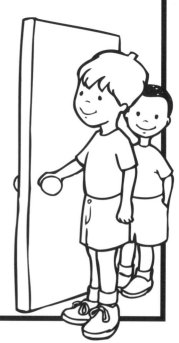

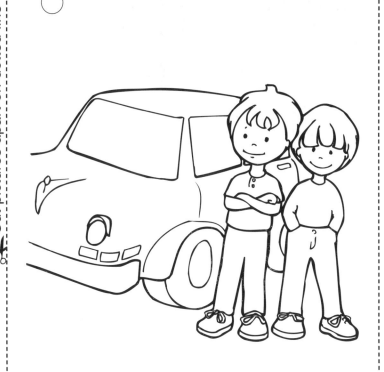

The boys are **beside** the car.

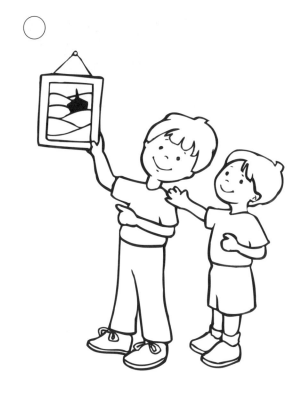

The boys are **beside** the picture.

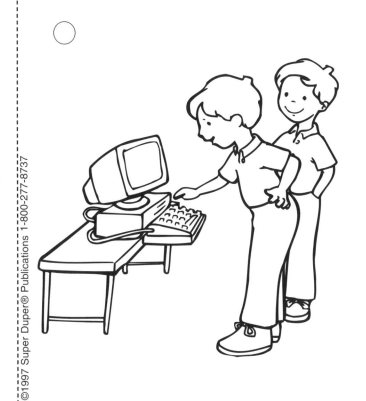

The boys are **beside** the computer.

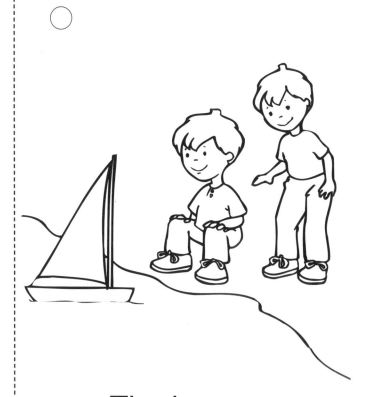

The boys are **beside** the boat.

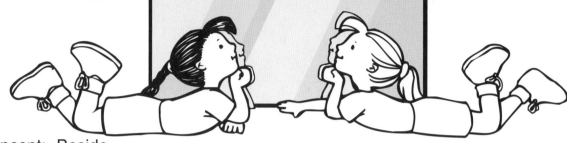

Concept: Beside

Date: _____

Ask your child to listen carefully as you read the following list of sentences slowly and clearly. It is important that your child not repeat the sentences but just listen to them quietly. Please spend one to two minutes daily reading these sentences to your child. After listening to these sentences, your child may color the pictures on the page!

1. The girls are beside the store.
2. The girls are beside the seesaw.
3. The girls are beside the snowman.
4. The girls are beside the wagon.
5. The girls are beside the mirror.

6. The girls are beside the bicycle.
7. The girls are beside the wheelchair.
8. The girls are beside the crib.
9. The girls are beside the suitcase.
10. The girls are beside the closet.

Additional Comments/Helpful Hints:

_____

_____

_____

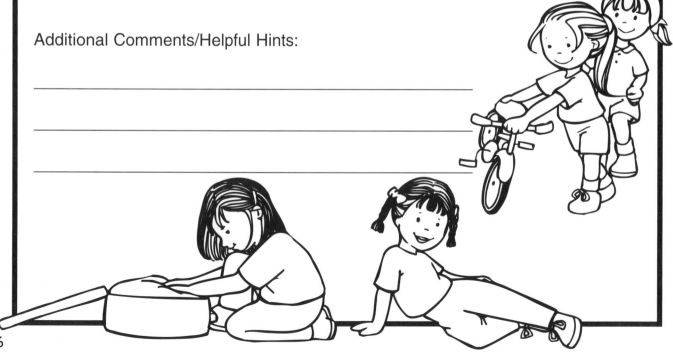

©1997 Super Duper® Publications 1-800-277-8737

The girls are **beside** the tree.

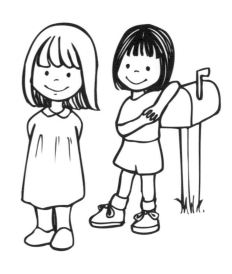

The girls are **beside** the mailbox.

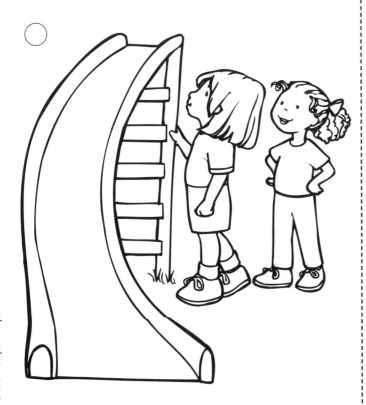

The girls are **beside** the slide.

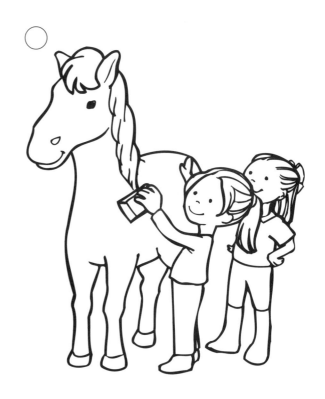

The girls are **beside** the horse.

167

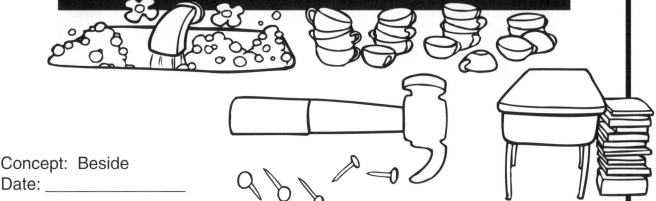

Concept: Beside

Date: _____

Ask your child to listen carefully as you read the following list of sentences slowly and clearly. It is important that your child not repeat the sentences but just listen to them quietly. Please spend one to two minutes daily reading these sentences to your child. After listening to these sentences, your child may color the pictures on the page!

1. The flowers are beside the vase.
2. The nails are beside the hammer.
3. The cups are beside the sink.
4. The monkeys are beside the tree.
5. The shoes are beside the door.
6. The puppies are beside the wagon.
7. The chairs are beside the window.
8. The horses are beside the gate.
9. The drums are beside the stage.
10. The books are beside the desk.

Additional Comments/Helpful Hints:

_____

_____

_____

©1997 Super Duper® Publications 1-800-277-8737

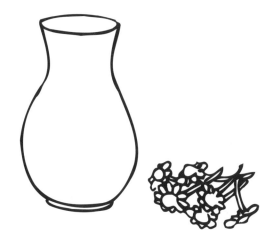

The flowers are **beside** the vase.

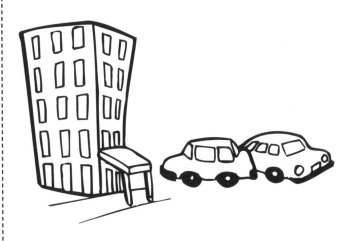

The cars are **beside** the building.

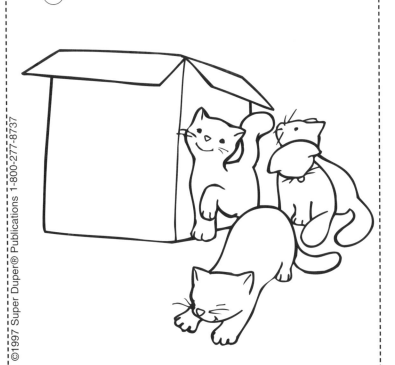

The kittens are **beside** the box.

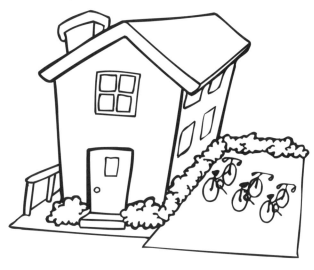

The bicycles are **beside** the house. 169

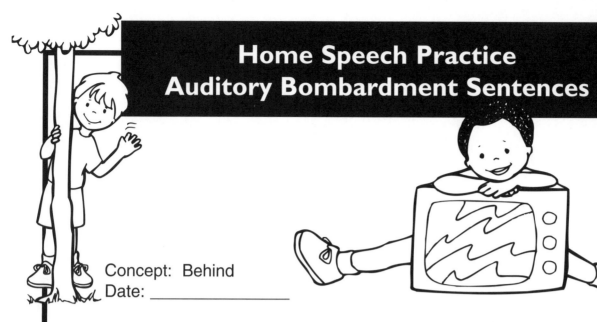

Home Speech Practice
Auditory Bombardment Sentences

Concept: Behind

Date: _____

Ask your child to listen carefully as you read the following list of sentences slowly and clearly. It is important that your child not repeat the sentences but just listen to them quietly. Please spend one to two minutes daily reading these sentences to your child. After listening to these sentences, your child may color the pictures on the page!

1. The boy is behind the tree.
2. The boy is behind the wagon.
3. The boy is behind the chair.
4. The boy is behind the couch.
5. The boy is behind the lamp.
6. The boy is behind the television.
7. The boy is behind the trumpet.
8. The boy is behind the slide.
9. The boy is behind the mailbox.
10. The boy is behind the gate.

Additional Comments/Helpful Hints:

_____

_____

_____

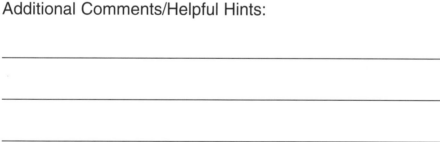

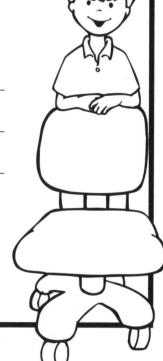

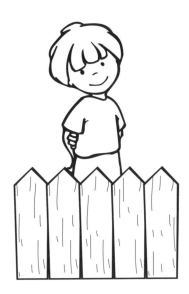

The boy is **behind** the fence.

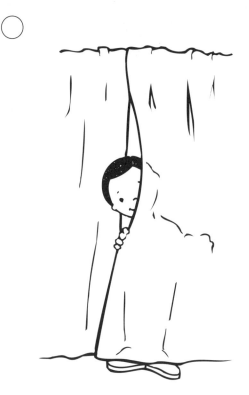

The boy is **behind** the curtains.

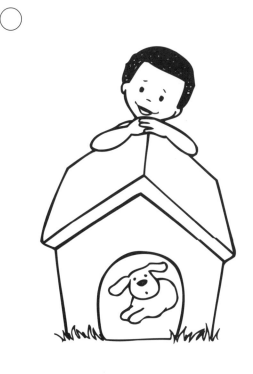

The boy is **behind** the doghouse.

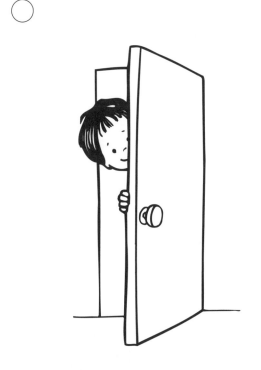

The boy is **behind** the door.

171

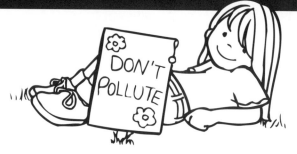

Home Speech Practice
Auditory Bombardment Sentences

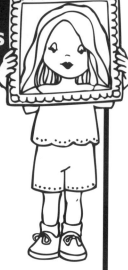

Concept: Behind

Date: _____

Ask your child to listen carefully as you read the following list of sentences slowly and clearly. It is important that your child not repeat the sentences but just listen to them quietly. Please spend one to two minutes daily reading these sentences to your child. After listening to these sentences, your child may color the pictures on the page!

1. The girl is behind the couch.
2. The girl is behind the building.
3. The girl is behind the picture.
4. The girl is behind the counter.
5. The girl is behind the ball.

6. The girl is behind the door.
7. The girl is behind the computer.
8. The girl is behind the bush.
9. The girl is behind the tractor.
10. The girl is behind the sign.

Additional Comments/Helpful Hints:

_____

_____

_____

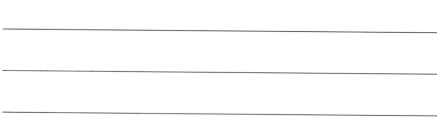

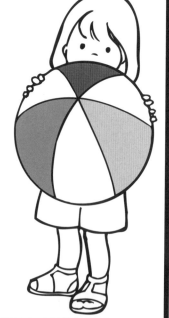

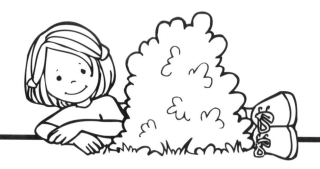

©1997 Super Duper® Publications 1-800-277-8737

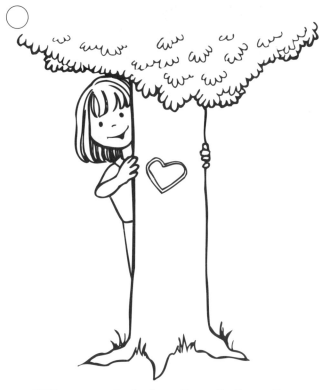

The girl is **behind** the tree.

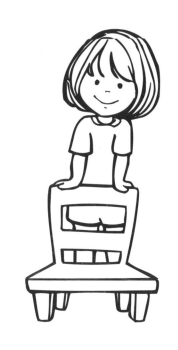

The girl is **behind** the chair.

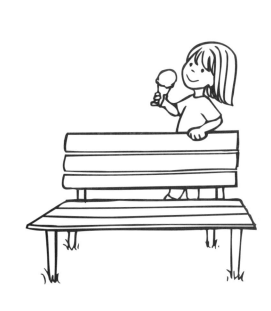

The girl is **behind** the bench.

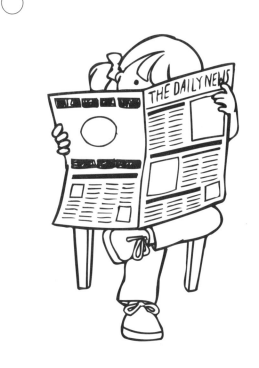

The girl is **behind** the newspaper.

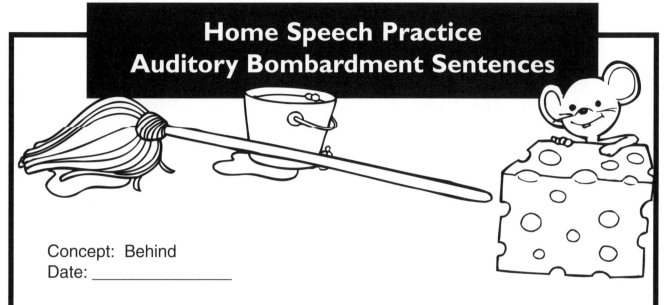

Home Speech Practice
Auditory Bombardment Sentences

Concept: Behind

Date: _____

Ask your child to listen carefully as you read the following list of sentences slowly and clearly. It is important that your child not repeat the sentences but just listen to them quietly. Please spend one to two minutes daily reading these sentences to your child. After listening to these sentences, your child may color the pictures on the page!

1. The ball is behind the fence.

2. The bucket is behind the mop.

3. The shoe is behind the couch.

4. The elephant is behind the house.

5. The car is behind the truck.

6. The dog is behind the door.

7. The snake is behind the rock.

8. The mouse is behind the cheese.

9. The chair is behind the desk.

10. The motorcycle is behind the car.

Additional Comments/Helpful Hints:

_____

_____

_____

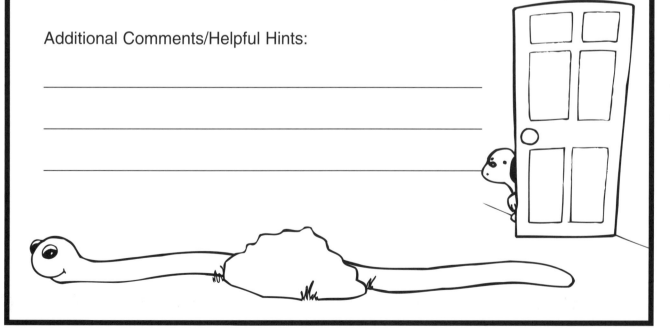

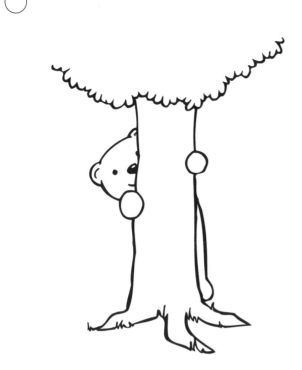

The bear is **behind** the tree.

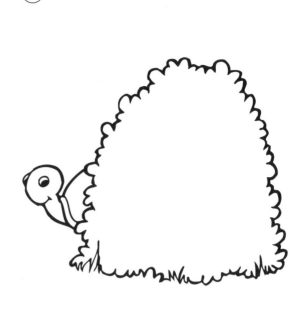

The turtle is **behind** the bush.

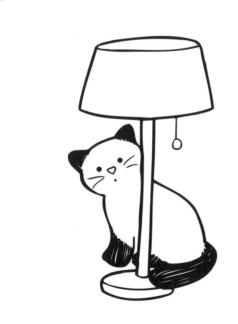

The cat is **behind** the lamp.

The worm is **behind** the apple.

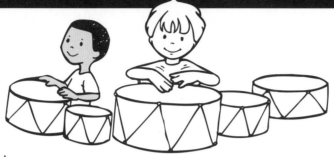

Home Speech Practice
Auditory Bombardment Sentences

Concept: Behind

Date: _____

Ask your child to listen carefully as you read the following list of sentences slowly and clearly. It is important that your child not repeat the sentences but just listen to them quietly. Please spend one to two minutes daily reading these sentences to your child. After listening to these sentences, your child may color the pictures on the page!

1. The boys are behind the cactus.
2. The boys are behind the tractor.
3. The boys are behind the flagpole.
4. The boys are behind the tent.
5. The boys are behind the box.
6. The boys are behind the drums.
7. The boys are behind the easel.
8. The boys are behind the newspaper.
9. The boys are behind the building.
10. The boys are behind the shopping cart.

Additional Comments/Helpful Hints:

_____

_____

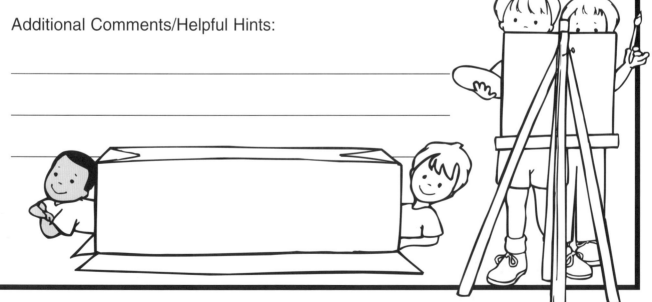

©1997 Super Duper® Publications 1-800-277-8737

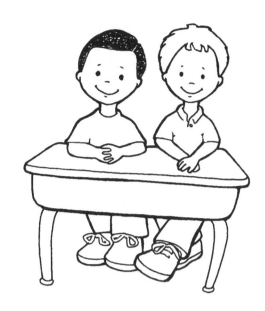

The boys are **behind** the desk.

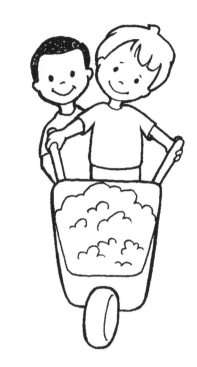

The boys are **behind** the wheelbarrow.

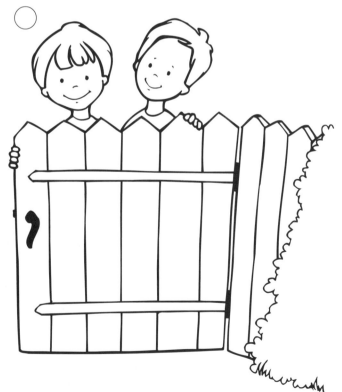

The boys are **behind** the gate.

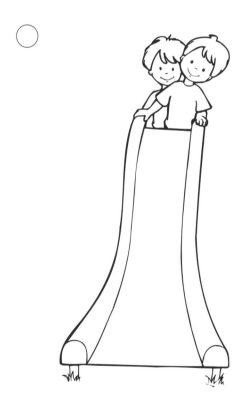

The boys are **behind** the slide.

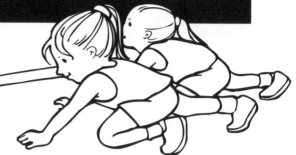

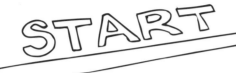

Concept: Behind

Date: _____

Ask your child to listen carefully as you read the following list of sentences slowly and clearly. It is important that your child not repeat the sentences but just listen to them quietly. Please spend one to two minutes daily reading these sentences to your child. After listening to these sentences, your child may color the pictures on the page!

1. The girls are behind the mailbox.
2. The girls are behind the horse.
3. The girls are behind the couch.
4. The girls are behind the scarecrow.
5. The girls are behind the line.

6. The girls are behind the microphone.
7. The girls are behind the barbecue.
8. The girls are behind the vacuum.
9. The girls are behind the flagpole.
10. The girls are behind the trailer.

Additional Comments/Helpful Hints:

_____

_____

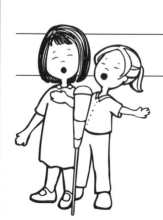

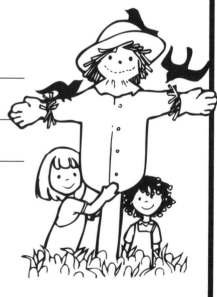

©1997 Super Duper® Publications 1-800-277-8737

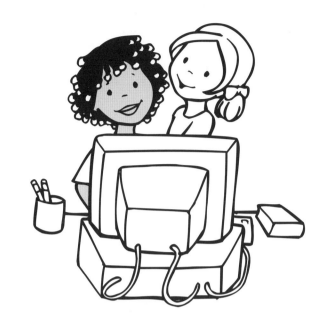

The girls are
behind the computer.

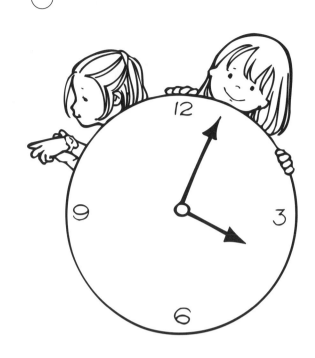

The girls are
behind the clock.

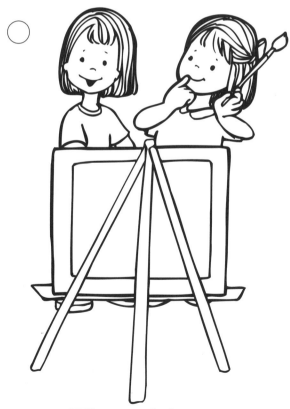

The girls are
behind the easel.

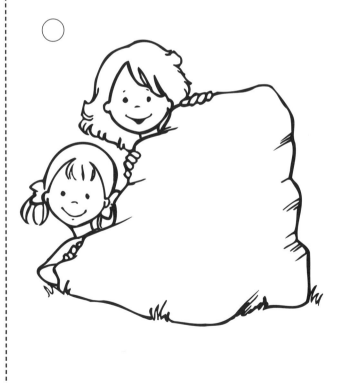

The girls are
behind the rock.

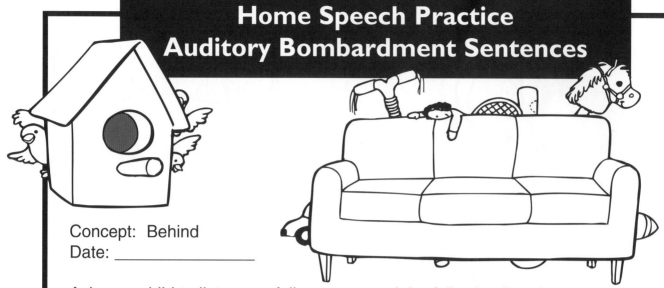

Home Speech Practice
Auditory Bombardment Sentences

Concept: Behind

Date: _____

Ask your child to listen carefully as you read the following list of sentences slowly and clearly. It is important that your child not repeat the sentences but just listen to them quietly. Please spend one to two minutes daily reading these sentences to your child. After listening to these sentences, your child may color the pictures on the page!

1. The birds are behind the birdhouse.

2. The pencils are behind the stapler.

3. The horses are behind the fence.

4. The backpacks are behind the door.

5. The cats are behind the car.

6. The rabbits are behind the carrots.

7. The ants are behind the picnic basket.

8. The snails are behind the plant.

9. The toys are behind the couch.

10. The chairs are behind the stage.

Additional Comments/Helpful Hints:

_____

_____

_____

©1997 Super Duper® Publications 1-800-277-8737

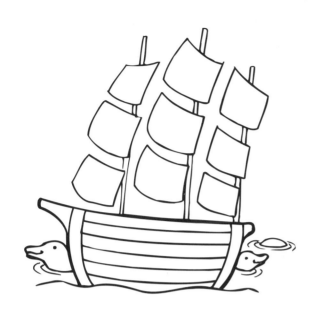

The dolphins are **behind** the ship.

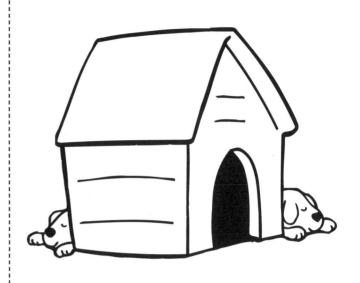

The dogs are **behind** the doghouse.

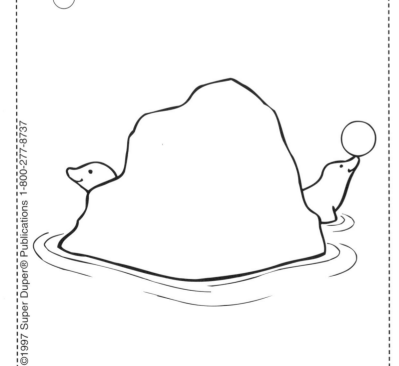

The seals are **behind** the rock.

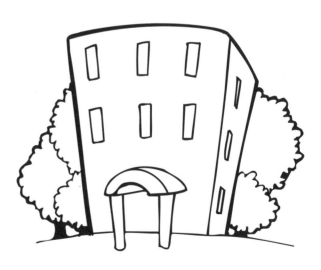

The trees are **behind** the building.

Home Speech Practice
Auditory Bombardment Sentences

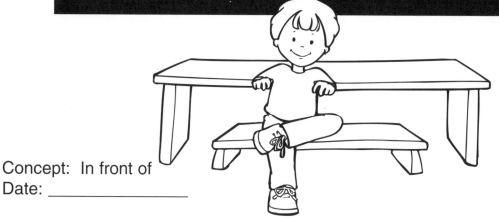

Concept: In front of

Date: _____

Ask your child to listen carefully as you read the following list of sentences slowly and clearly. It is important that your child not repeat the sentences but just listen to them quietly. Please spend one to two minutes daily reading these sentences to your child. After listening to these sentences, your child may color the pictures on the page!

1. The boy is in front of the bicycle.
2. The boy is in front of the tree.
3. The boy is in front of the wagon.
4. The boy is in front of the desk.
5. The boy is in front of the flag.

6. The boy is in front of the ball.
7. The boy is in front of the door.
8. The boy is in front of the chair.
9. The boy is in front of the truck.
10. The boy is in front of the table.

Additional Comments/Helpful Hints:

_____

_____

_____

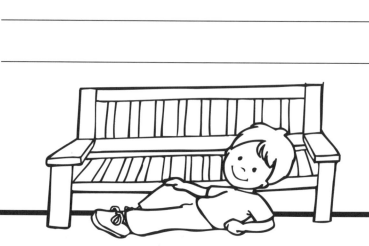

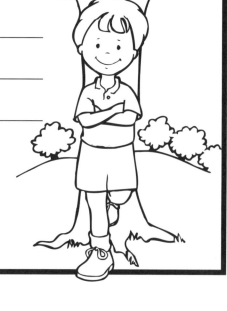

©1997 Super Duper® Publications 1-800-277-8737

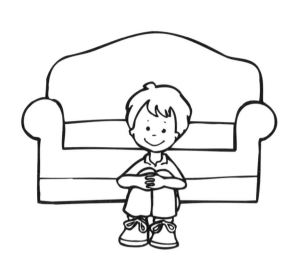

The boy is **in front of** the couch.

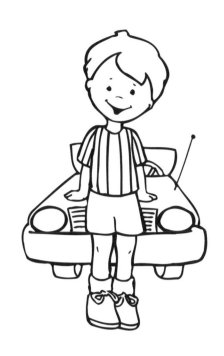

The boy is **in front of** the car.

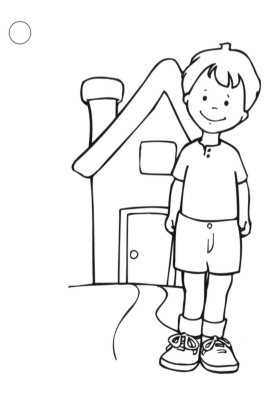

The boy is **in front of** the house.

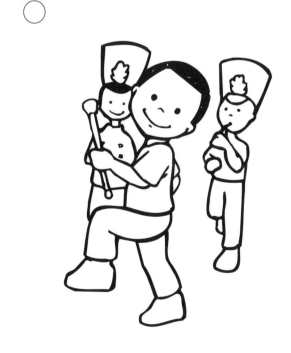

The boy is **in front of** the parade.

183

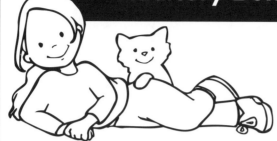

Home Speech Practice
Auditory Bombardment Sentences

Concept: In front of

Date: _____

Ask your child to listen carefully as you read the following list of sentences slowly and clearly. It is important that your child not repeat the sentences but just listen to them quietly. Please spend one to two minutes daily reading these sentences to your child. After listening to these sentences, your child may color the pictures on the page!

1. The girl is in front of the mirror.

2. The girl is in front of the cat.

3. The girl is in front of the motorcycle.

4. The girl is in front of the bench.

5. The girl is in front of the clown.

6. The girl is in front of the swing.

7. The girl is in front of the line.

8. The girl is in front of the building.

9. The girl is in front of the chalkboard.

10. The girl is in front of the truck.

Additional Comments/Helpful Hints:

_____

_____

_____

184

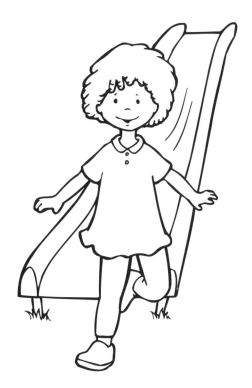

The girl is **in front of** the slide.

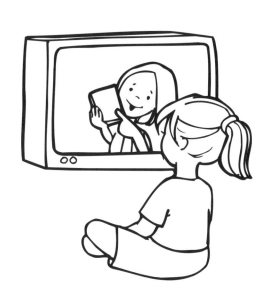

The girl is **in front of** the television.

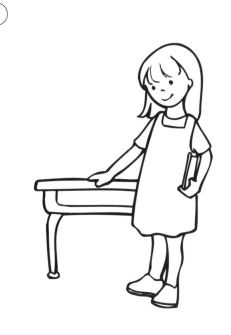

The girl is **in front of** the desk.

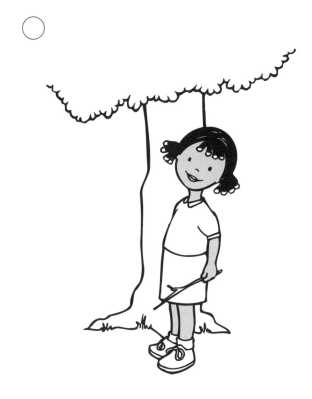

The girl is **in front of** the tree.

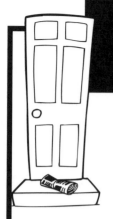

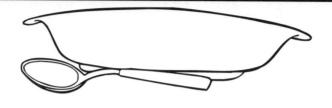

Home Speech Practice
Auditory Bombardment Sentences

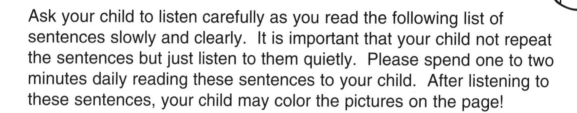

Concept: In front of

Date: _____

Ask your child to listen carefully as you read the following list of sentences slowly and clearly. It is important that your child not repeat the sentences but just listen to them quietly. Please spend one to two minutes daily reading these sentences to your child. After listening to these sentences, your child may color the pictures on the page!

1. The ball is in front of the tree.

2. The boat is in front of the bridge.

3. The dog is in front of the statue.

4. The newspaper is in front of the door.

5. The bear is in front of the tent.

6. The flower is in front of the window.

7. The spoon is in front of the bowl.

8. The car is in front of the garage.

9. The box is in front of the elephant.

10. The teddy bear is in front of the couch.

Additional Comments/Helpful Hints:

_____

_____

_____

©1997 Super Duper® Publications 1-800-277-8737

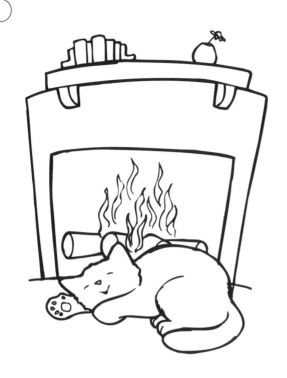

The cat is **in front of** the fireplace.

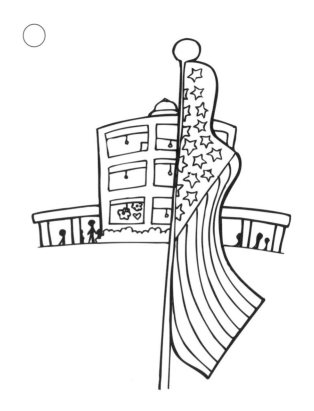

The flag is **in front of** the school.

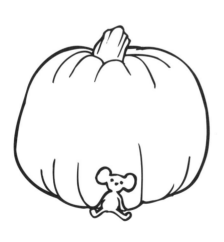

The mouse is **in front of** the pumpkin.

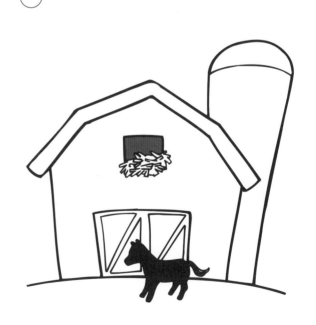

The horse is **in front of** the barn.

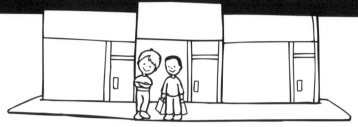

Home Speech Practice
Auditory Bombardment Sentences

Concept: In front of

Date: _____

Ask your child to listen carefully as you read the following list of sentences slowly and clearly. It is important that your child not repeat the sentences but just listen to them quietly. Please spend one to two minutes daily reading these sentences to your child. After listening to these sentences, your child may color the pictures on the page!

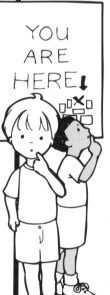

1. The boys are in front of the garage.

2. The boys are in front of the store.

3. The boys are in front of the fence.

4. The boys are in front of the zebra.

5. The boys are in front of the slide.

6. The boys are in front of the couch.

7. The boys are in front of the box.

8. The boys are in front of the stage.

9. The boys are in front of the sign.

10. The boys are in front of the clock.

Additional Comments/Helpful Hints:

_____

_____

_____

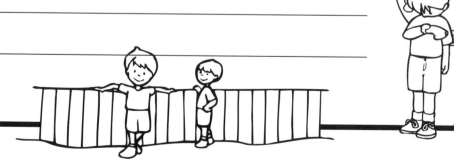

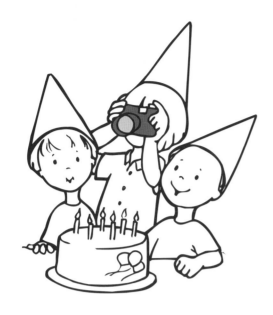

The boys are **in front of** the camera.

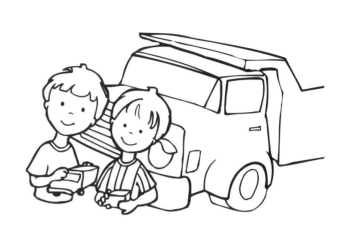

The boys are **in front of** the truck.

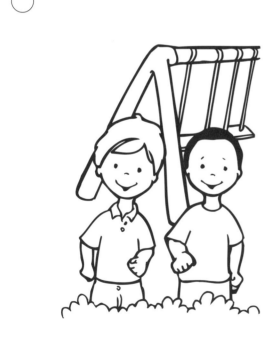

The boys are **in front of** the swings.

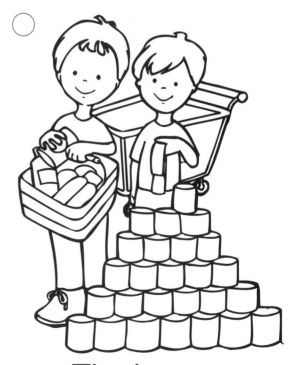

The boys are **in front of** the shopping cart.

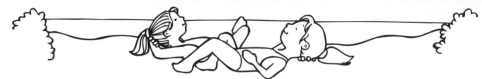

Home Speech Practice
Auditory Bombardment Sentences

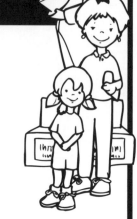

Concept: In front of

Date: _____

Ask your child to listen carefully as you read the following list of sentences slowly and clearly. It is important that your child not repeat the sentences but just listen to them quietly. Please spend one to two minutes daily reading these sentences to your child. After listening to these sentences, your child may color the pictures on the page!

1. The girls are in front of the gate.

2. The girls are in front of the bookshelf.

3. The girls are in front of the picnic table.

4. The girls are in front of the tepee.

5. The girls are in front of the ship.

6. The girls are in front of the lake.

7. The girls are in front of the stairs.

8. The girls are in front of the television.

9. The girls are in front of the wagon.

10. The girls are in front of the statue.

Additional Comments/Helpful Hints:

_____

_____

_____

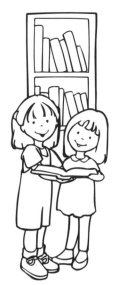

©1997 Super Duper® Publications 1-800-277-8737

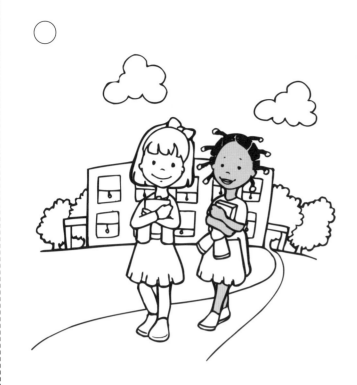

The girls are **in front of** the school.

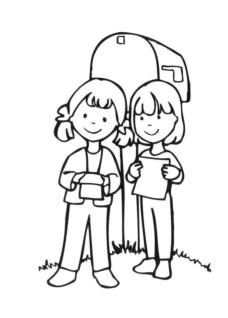

The girls are **in front of** the mailbox.

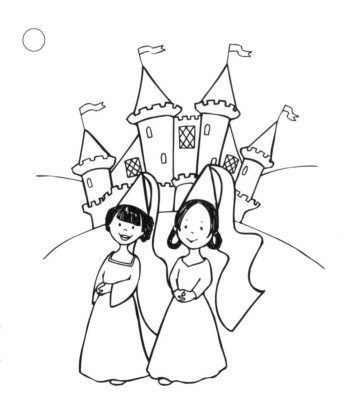

The girls are **in front of** the castle.

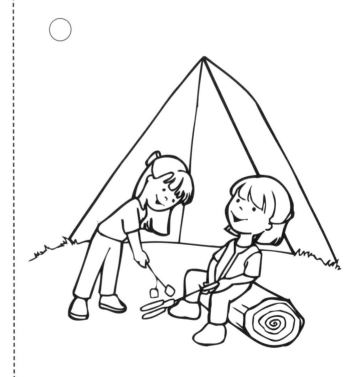

The girls are **in front of** the tent.

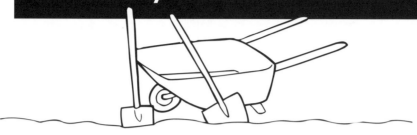

Home Speech Practice
Auditory Bombardment Sentences

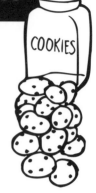

Concept: In front of

Date: _____

Ask your child to listen carefully as you read the following list of sentences slowly and clearly. It is important that your child not repeat the sentences but just listen to them quietly. Please spend one to two minutes daily reading these sentences to your child. After listening to these sentences, your child may color the pictures on the page!

1. The elephants are in front of the parade.
2. The shovels are in front of the wheelbarrow.
3. The books are in front of the classroom.
4. The coins are in front of the pirate.
5. The clothes are in front of the basket.
6. The boots are in front of the closet.
7. The crayons are in front of the paper.
8. The skates are in front of the door.
9. The cookies are in front of the jar.
10. The soldiers are in front of the building.

Additional Comments/Helpful Hints:

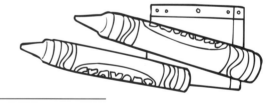

_____

_____

_____

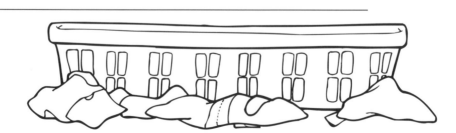

192

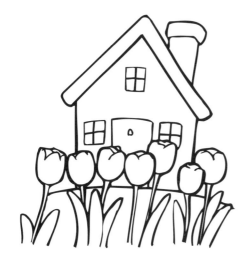

The flowers are **in front of** the house.

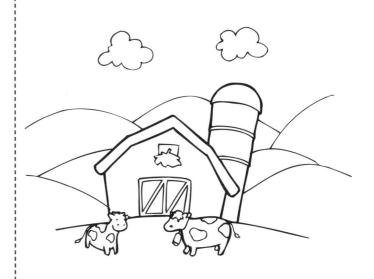

The cows are **in front of** the barn.

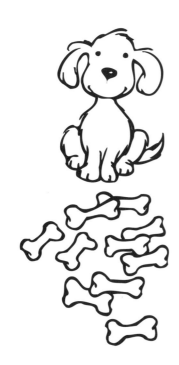

The bones are **in front of** the dog.

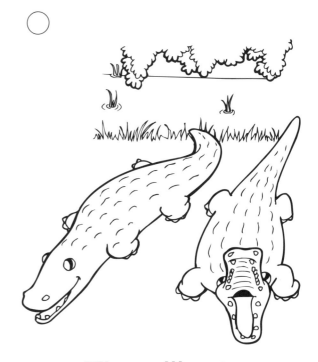

The alligators are **in front of** the swamp.

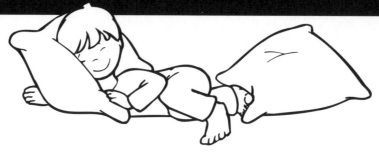

Home Speech Practice
Auditory Bombardment Sentences

Concept: Between

Date: _____

Ask your child to listen carefully as you read the following list of sentences slowly and clearly. It is important that your child not repeat the sentences but just listen to them quietly. Please spend one to two minutes daily reading these sentences to your child. After listening to these sentences, your child may color the pictures on the page!

1. The boy is between the bicycles.
2. The boy is between the swings.
3. The boy is between the poles.
4. The boy is between the trees.
5. The boy is between the slides.

6. The boy is between the pillows.
7. The boy is between the dogs.
8. The boy is between the suitcases.
9. The boy is between the tents.
10. The boy is between the cars.

Additional Comments/Helpful Hints:

_____

_____

_____

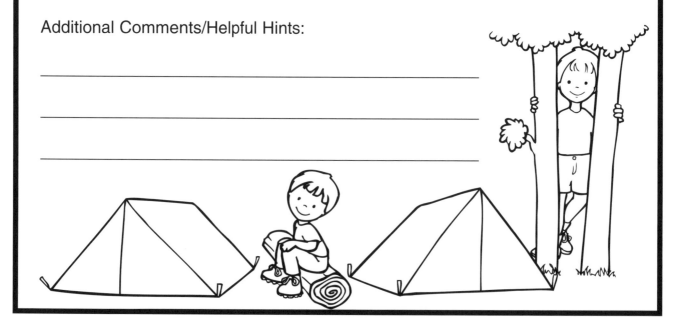

194

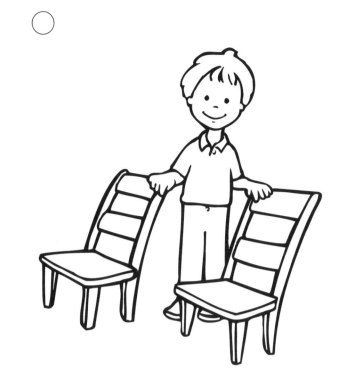

The boy is **between** the chairs.

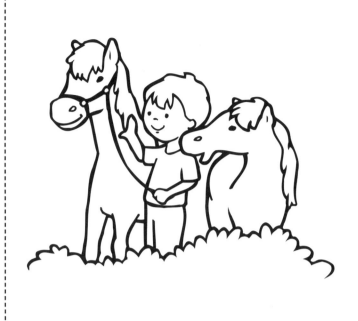

The boy is **between** the horses.

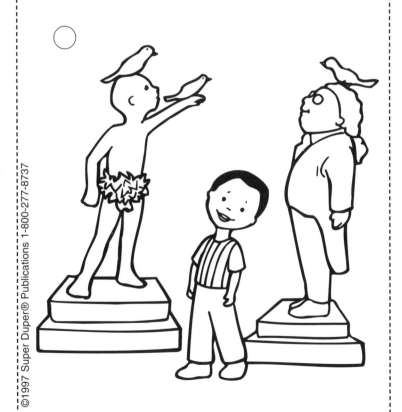

The boy is **between** the statues.

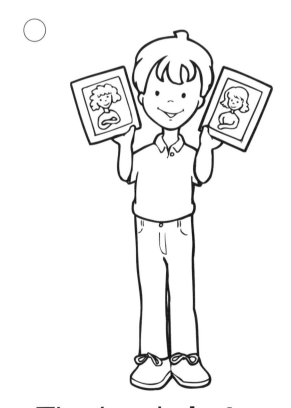

The boy is **between** the pictures.

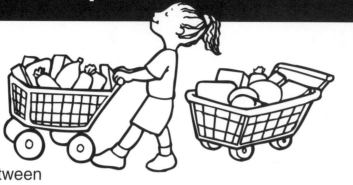

Home Speech Practice
Auditory Bombardment Sentences

Concept: Between

Date: _____

Ask your child to listen carefully as you read the following list of sentences slowly and clearly. It is important that your child not repeat the sentences but just listen to them quietly. Please spend one to two minutes daily reading these sentences to your child. After listening to these sentences, your child may color the pictures on the page!

1. The girl is between the lights.
2. The girl is between the benches.
3. The girl is between the desks.
4. The girl is between the buses.
5. The girl is between the towels.

6. The girl is between the flowers.
7. The girl is between the boxes.
8. The girl is between the cats.
9. The girl is between the shopping carts.
10. The girl is between the lines.

Additional Comments/Helpful Hints:

_____

_____

_____

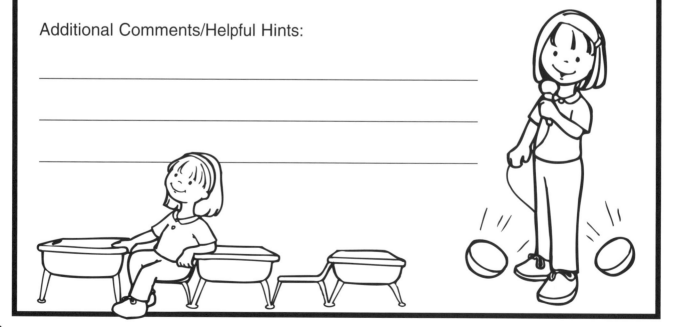

©1997 Super Duper® Publications 1-800-277-8737

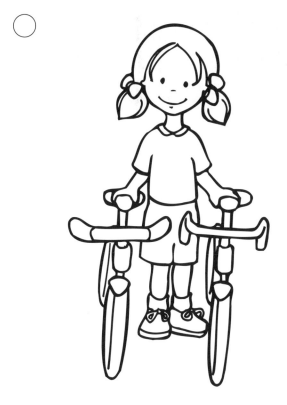

The girl is **between** the bicycles.

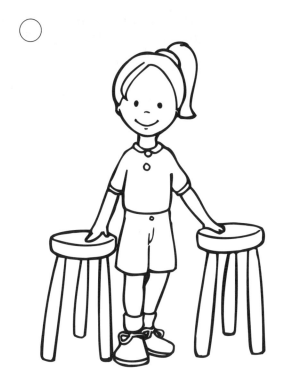

The girl is **between** the stools.

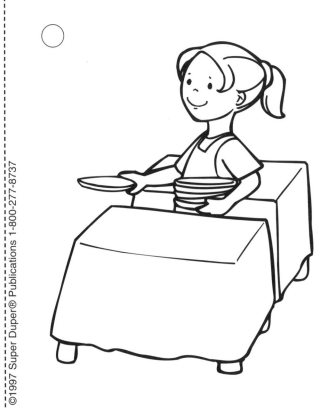

The girl is **between** the tables.

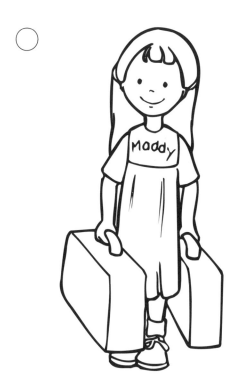

The girl is **between** the suitcases.

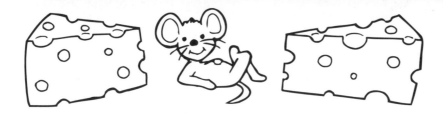
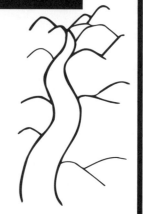

Concept: Between

Date: _____

Ask your child to listen carefully as you read the following list of sentences slowly and clearly. It is important that your child not repeat the sentences but just listen to them quietly. Please spend one to two minutes daily reading these sentences to your child. After listening to these sentences, your child may color the pictures on the page!

1. The car is between the lines.

2. The table is between the chairs.

3. The plate is between the cups.

4. The bed is between the bookcases.

5. The flower is between the bushes.

6. The motorcycle is between the cars.

7. The sandbox is between the swings.

8. The river is between the mountains.

9. The clock is between the chalk boards.

10. The mouse is between the slices of cheese.

Additional Comments/Helpful Hints:

_____

_____

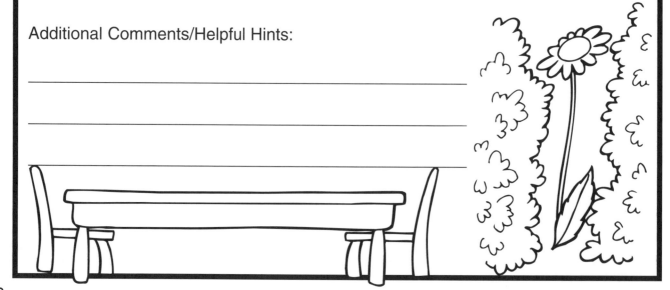

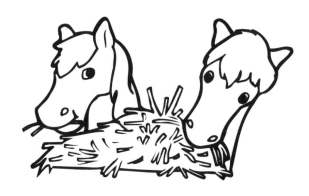

The hay is **between** the horses.

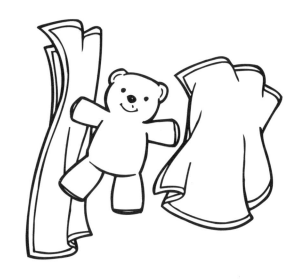

The teddy bear is **between** the blankets.

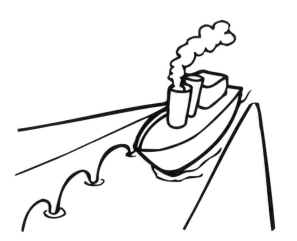

The ship is **between** the bridges.

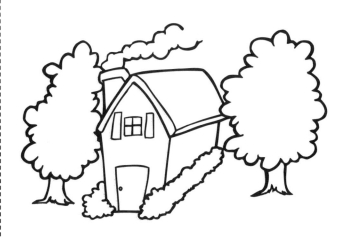

The house is **between** the trees.

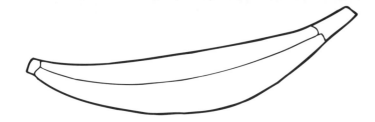

Concept: Whole

Date: _____

Ask your child to listen carefully as you read the following list of sentences slowly and clearly. It is important that your child not repeat the sentences but just listen to them quietly. Please spend one to two minutes daily reading these sentences to your child. After listening to these sentences, your child may color the pictures on the page!

1. This is a whole banana.
2. This is a whole pickle.
3. This is a whole potato.
4. This is a whole cupcake.
5. This is a whole orange.

6. This is a whole grapefruit.
7. This is a whole popsicle.
8. This is a whole cantaloupe.
9. This is a whole bagel.
10. This is a whole glass of milk.

Additional Comments/Helpful Hints:

_____

_____

_____

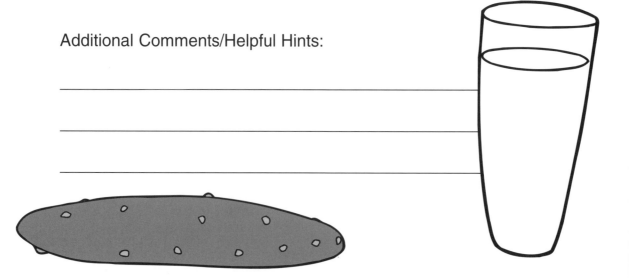

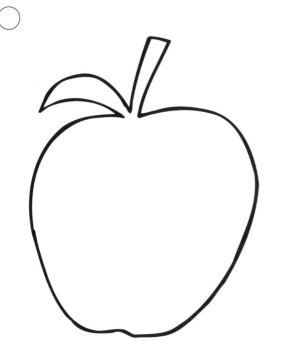

This is a **whole** apple.

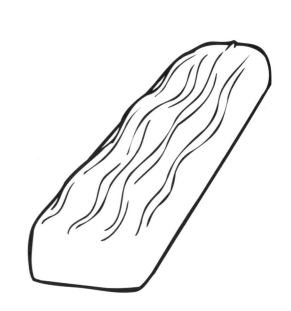

This is a **whole** candy bar.

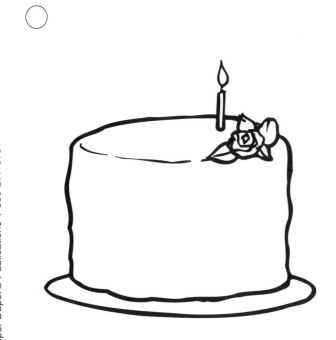

This is a **whole** cake.

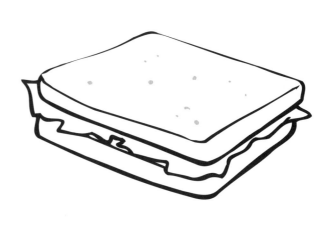

This is a **whole** sandwich.

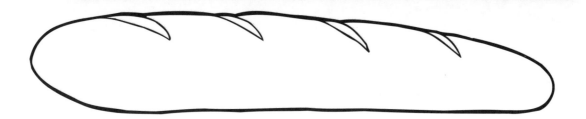

Concept: Whole

Date: _____

Ask your child to listen carefully as you read the following list of sentences slowly and clearly. It is important that your child not repeat the sentences but just listen to them quietly. Please spend one to two minutes daily reading these sentences to your child. After listening to these sentences, your child may color the pictures on the page!

1. This is a whole tomato.

2. This is a whole onion.

3. This is a whole pumpkin.

4. This is a whole muffin.

5. This is a whole peach.

6. This is a whole pear.

7. This is a whole hot dog.

8. This is a whole pineapple.

9. This is a whole loaf of bread.

10. This is a whole hamburger.

Additional Comments/Helpful Hints:

_____

_____

_____

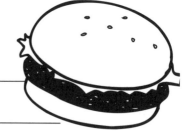

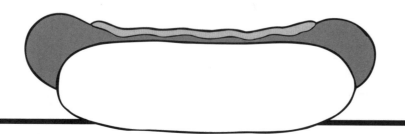

©1997 Super Duper® Publications 1-800-277-8737

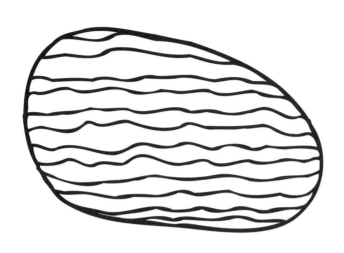

This is a **whole** watermelon.

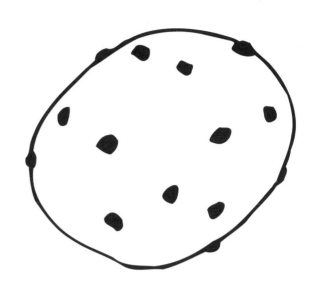

This is a **whole** cookie.

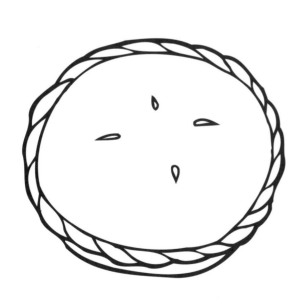

This is a **whole** pie.

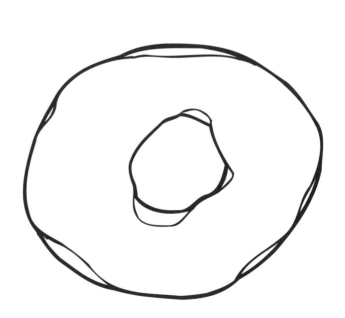

This is a **whole** donut.

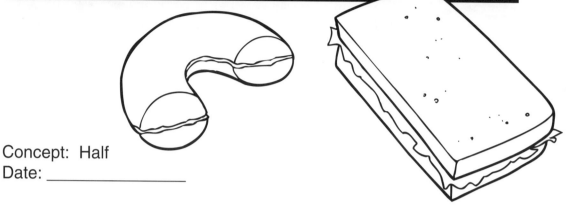

Home Speech Practice
Auditory Bombardment Sentences

Concept: Half

Date: _____

Ask your child to listen carefully as you read the following list of sentences slowly and clearly. It is important that your child not repeat the sentences but just listen to them quietly. Please spend one to two minutes daily reading these sentences to your child. After listening to these sentences, your child may color the pictures on the page!

1. This is half of a sandwich.
2. This is half of a peach.
3. This is half of a tomato.
4. This is half of a cookie.
5. This is half of a pickle.

6. This is half of a glass of milk.
7. This is half of a cherry.
8. This is half of a candy bar.
9. This is half of a pancake.
10. This is half of a strawberry.

Additional Comments/Helpful Hints:

_____

_____

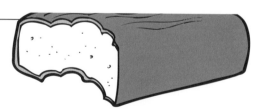

©1997 Super Duper® Publications 1-800-277-8737

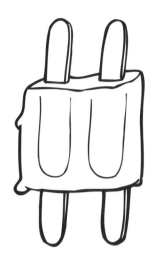

This is **half** of
a popscicle.

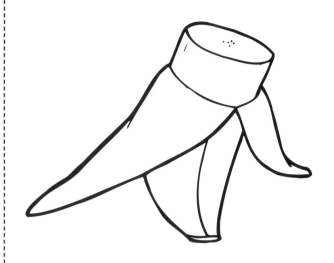

This is **half**
of a banana.

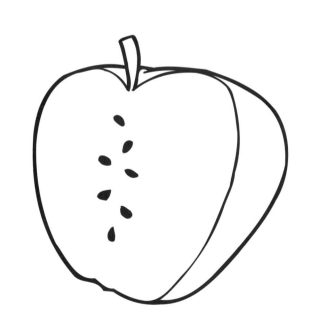

This is **half** of an apple.

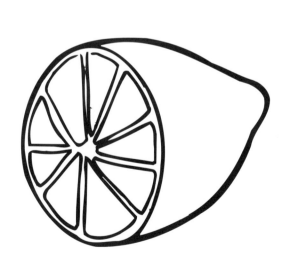

This is **half**
of a lemon.

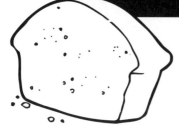
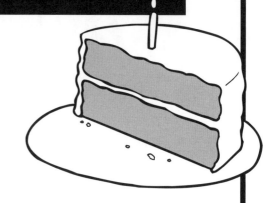

Concept: Half

Date: _____

Ask your child to listen carefully as you read the following list of sentences slowly and clearly. It is important that your child not repeat the sentences but just listen to them quietly. Please spend one to two minutes daily reading these sentences to your child. After listening to these sentences, your child may color the pictures on the page!

1. This is half of a donut.

2. This is half of a bagel.

3. This is half of a muffin.

4. This is half of a burrito.

5. This is half of a cake.

6. This is half of a pear.

7. This is half of a biscuit.

8. This is half of a pineapple.

9. This is half of an onion.

10. This is half of a grapefruit.

Additional Comments/Helpful Hints:

_____

_____

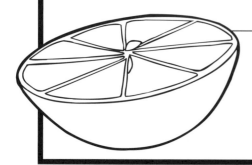
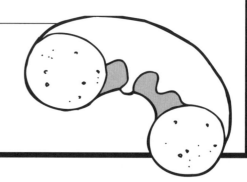

©1997 Super Duper® Publications 1-800-277-8737

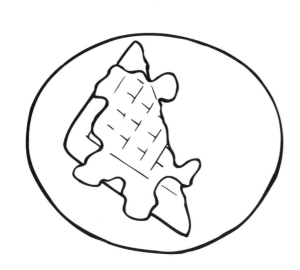

This is **half** of a waffle.

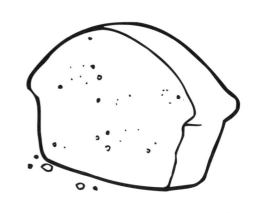

This is **half** of a cupcake.

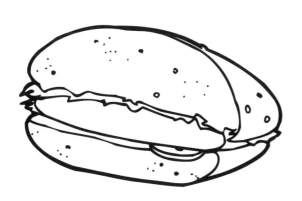

This is **half** of a hamburger.

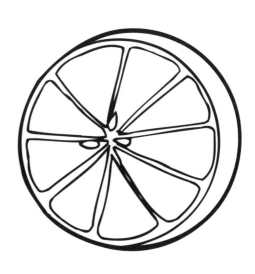

This is **half** of an orange.

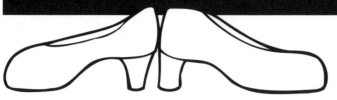

Home Speech Practice
Auditory Bombardment Sentences

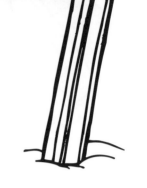

Concept: Pair

Date: _____

Ask your child to listen carefully as you read the following list of sentences slowly and clearly. It is important that your child not repeat the sentences but just listen to them quietly. Please spend one to two minutes daily reading these sentences to your child. After listening to these sentences, your child may color the pictures on the page!

1. This is a pair of shoes.
2. This is a pair of candles.
3. This is a pair of batteries.
4. This is a pair of pants.
5. This is a pair of gloves.

6. This is a pair of sandals.
7. This is a pair of monkeys.
8. This is a pair of roller blades.
9. This is a pair of elephants.
10. This is a pair of skis.

Additional Comments/Helpful Hints:

_____

_____

_____

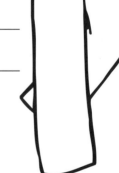

208

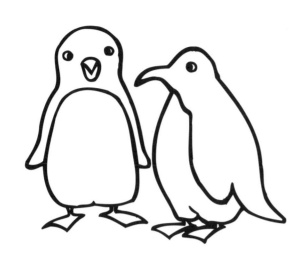

This is a **pair** of penguins.

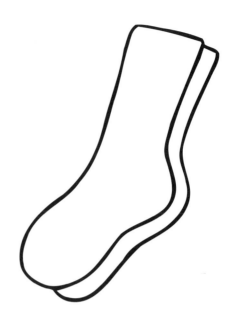

This is a **pair** of socks.

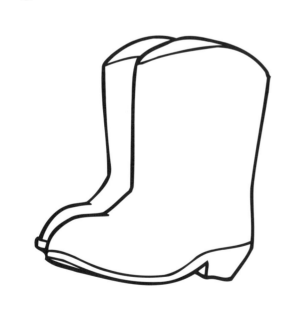

This is a **pair** of boots.

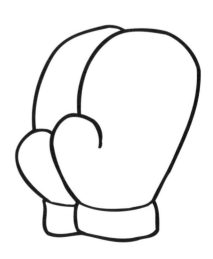

This is a **pair** of mittens.

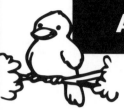

 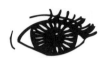 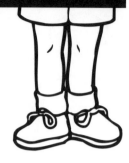

Concept: Pair

Date: _____

Ask your child to listen carefully as you read the following list of sentences slowly and clearly. It is important that your child not repeat the sentences but just listen to them quietly. Please spend one to two minutes daily reading these sentences to your child. After listening to these sentences, your child may color the pictures on the page!

1. This is a pair of buttons.

2. This is a pair of earmuffs.

3. This is a pair of knitting needles.

4. This is a pair of birds.

5. This is a pair of scissors.

6. This is a pair of eyes.

7. This is a pair of cats.

8. This is a pair of glasses.

9. This is a pair of legs.

10. This is a pair of shorts.

Additional Comments/Helpful Hints:

_____

_____

_____

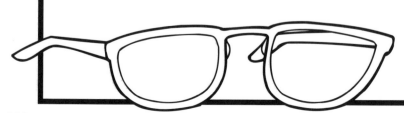 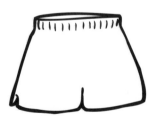

©1997 Super Duper® Publications 1-800-277-8737

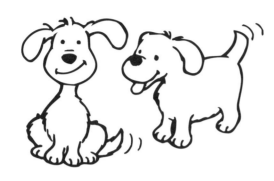

This is a **pair** of dogs.

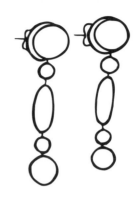

This is a **pair** of earrings.

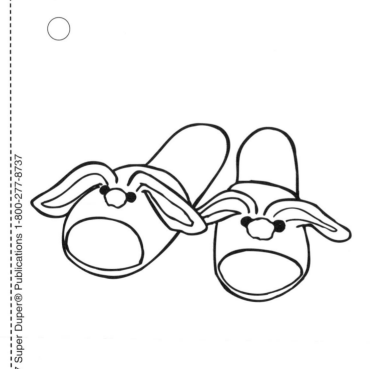

This is a **pair** of slippers.

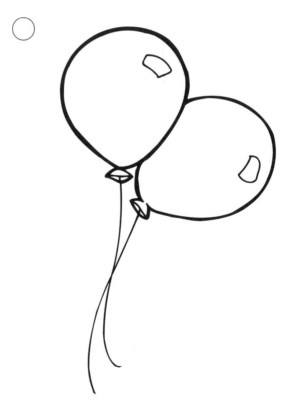

This is a **pair** of balloons.

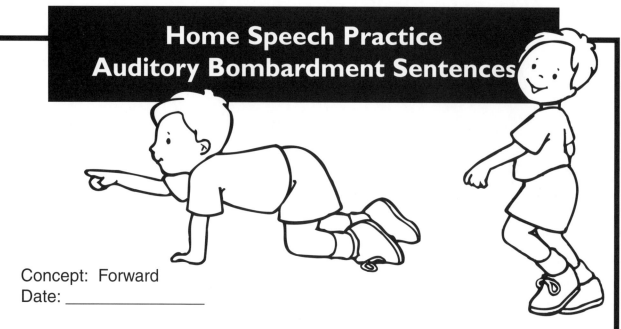

Home Speech Practice
Auditory Bombardment Sentences

Concept: Forward

Date: _____

Ask your child to listen carefully as you read the following list of sentences slowly and clearly. It is important that your child not repeat the sentences but just listen to them quietly. Please spend one to two minutes daily reading these sentences to your child. After listening to these sentences, your child may color the pictures on the page!

1. The boy is hopping forward.
2. The boy is swimming forward.
3. The boy is leaning forward.
4. The boy is pointing forward.
5. The boy is dancing forward.
6. The boy is leaping forward.
7. The boy is kicking forward.
8. The boy is jogging forward.
9. The boy is pushing forward.
10. The boy is skipping forward.

Additional Comments/Helpful Hints:

_____

_____

_____

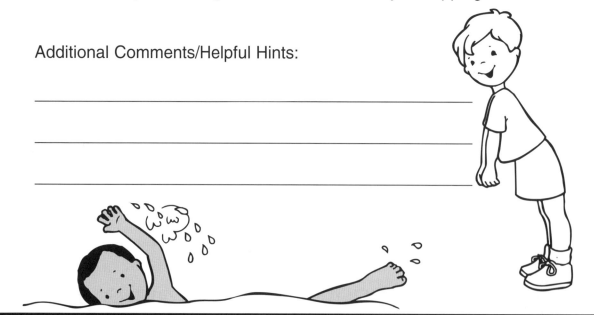

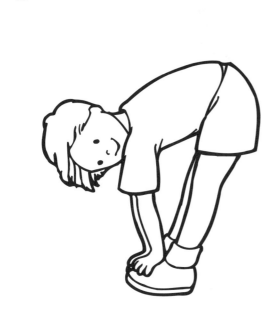

The boy is
bending **forward**.

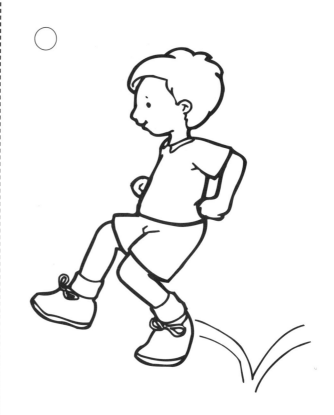

The boy is
jumping **forward**.

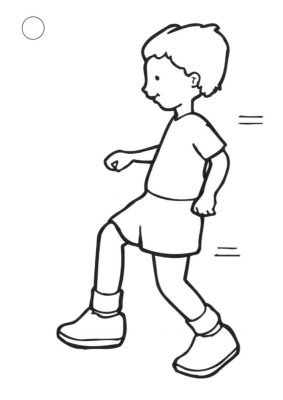

The boy is
running **forward**.

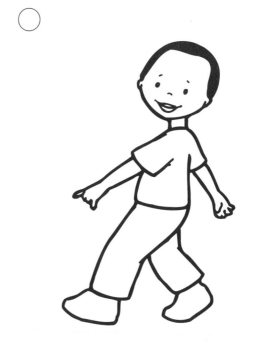

The boy is
walking **forward**. 213

Home Speech Practice
Auditory Bombardment Sentences

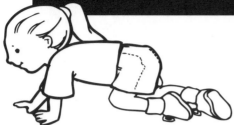

Concept: Forward
Date: _____

Ask your child to listen carefully as you read the following list of sentences slowly and clearly. It is important that your child not repeat the sentences but just listen to them quietly. Please spend one to two minutes daily reading these sentences to your child. After listening to these sentences, your child may color the pictures on the page!

1. The girl is riding forward.
2. The girl is sliding forward.
3. The girl is jumping forward.
4. The girl is skiing forward.
5. The girl is bending forward.
6. The girl is swinging forward.
7. The girl is crawling forward.
8. The girl is going forward.
9. The girl is throwing forward.
10. The girl is skipping forward.

Additional Comments/Helpful Hints:

_____

_____

_____

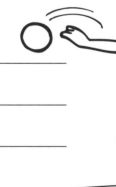

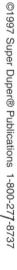
©1997 Super Duper® Publications 1-800-277-8737

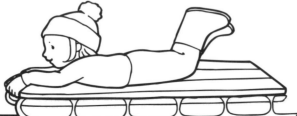

214

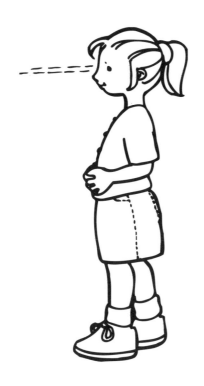

The girl is
looking **forward**.

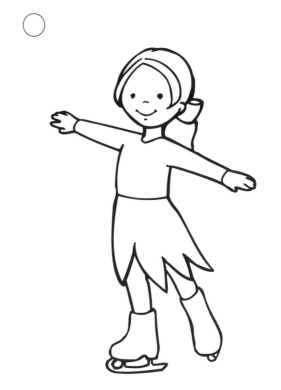

The girl is
skating **forward**.

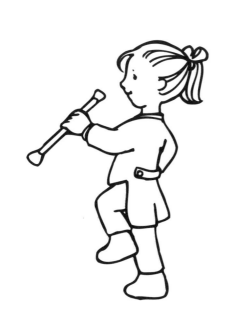

The girl is
marching **forward**.

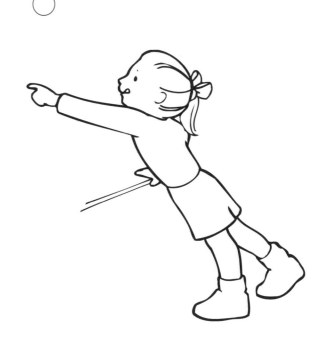

The girl is reaching
forward.

215

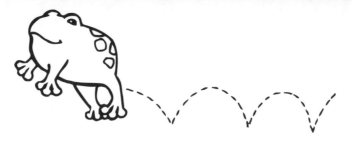

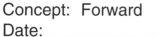

Concept: Forward

Date: _____

Ask your child to listen carefully as you read the following list of sentences slowly and clearly. It is important that your child not repeat the sentences but just listen to them quietly. Please spend one to two minutes daily reading these sentences to your child. After listening to these sentences, your child may color the pictures on the page!

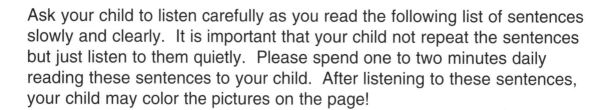

1. The kangaroo is hopping forward.

2. The lion is running forward.

3. The frog is jumping forward.

4. The giraffe is leaning forward.

5. The cat is looking forward.

6. The fish is swimming forward.

7. The bear is moving forward.

8. The monkey is swinging forward.

9. The ball is rolling forward.

10. The horse is galloping forward.

Additional Comments/Helpful Hints:

_____

_____

_____

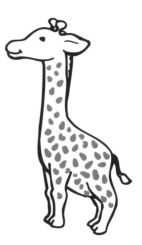

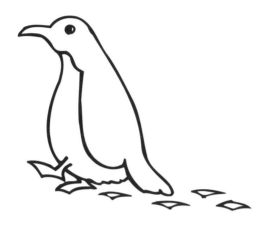

The penguin is
walking **forward**.

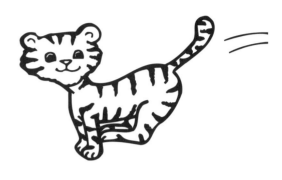

The tiger is
running **forward**.

©1997 Super Duper® Publications 1-800-277-8737

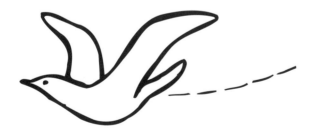

The bird is
flying **forward**.

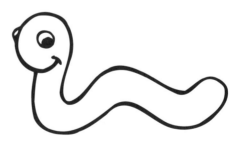

The caterpillar
is crawling
forward.

217

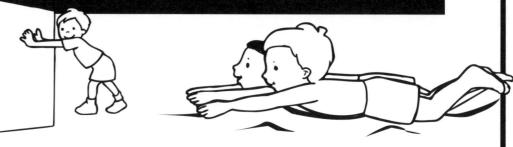

Home Speech Practice
Auditory Bombardment Sentences

Concept: Forward

Date: _____

Ask your child to listen carefully as you read the following list of sentences slowly and clearly. It is important that your child not repeat the sentences but just listen to them quietly. Please spend one to two minutes daily reading these sentences to your child. After listening to these sentences, your child may color the pictures on the page!

1. The boys are sledding forward.
2. The boys are marching forward.
3. The boys are leaning forward.
4. The boys are skipping forward.
5. The boys are swimming forward.
6. The boys are bending forward.
7. The boys are diving forward.
8. The boys are jumping forward.
9. The boys are moving forward.
10. The boys are sitting forward.

Additional Comments/Helpful Hints:

_____

_____

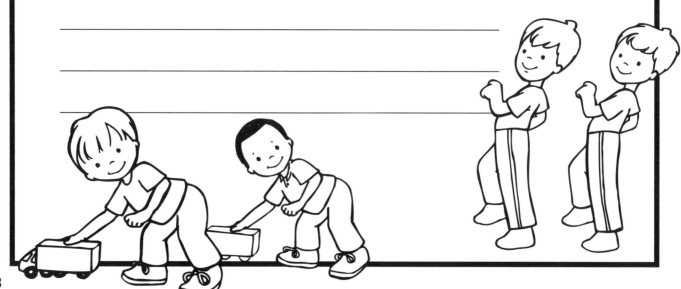

218

The boys are
crawling **forward**.

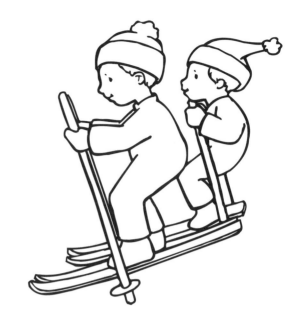

The boys are
skiing **forward**.

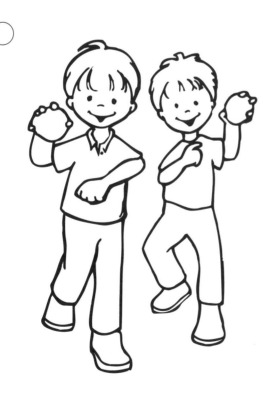

The boys are
throwing **forward**.

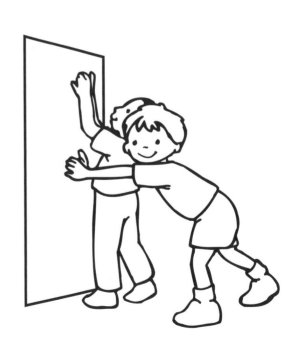

The boys are
pushing **forward**. 219

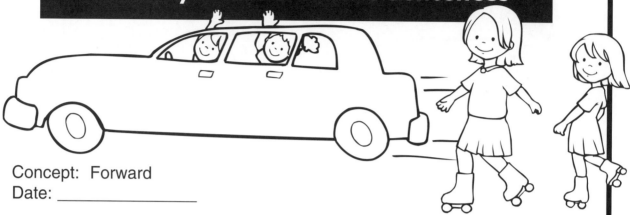

Home Speech Practice
Auditory Bombardment Sentences

Concept: Forward

Date: _____

Ask your child to listen carefully as you read the following list of sentences slowly and clearly. It is important that your child not repeat the sentences but just listen to them quietly. Please spend one to two minutes daily reading these sentences to your child. After listening to these sentences, your child may color the pictures on the page!

1. The girls are falling forward.

2. The girls are pointing forward.

3. The girls are riding forward.

4. The girls are looking forward.

5. The girls are reaching forward.

6. The girls are marching forward.

7. The girls are running forward.

8. The girls are hopping forward.

9. The girls are leaping forward.

10. The girls are skating forward.

Additional Comments/Helpful Hints:

_____

_____

_____

©1997 Super Duper® Publications 1-800-277-8737

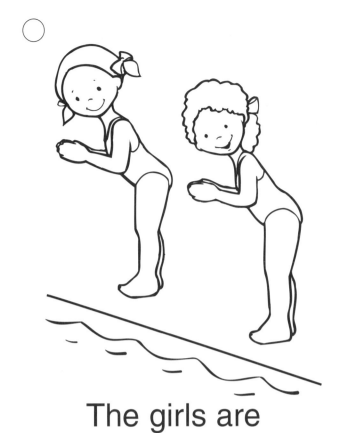

The girls are
diving **forward**.

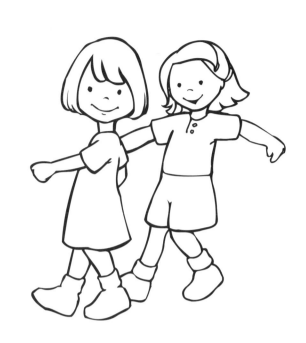

The girls are
walking **forward**.

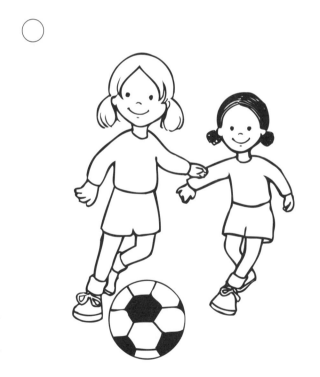

The girls are
kicking **forward**.

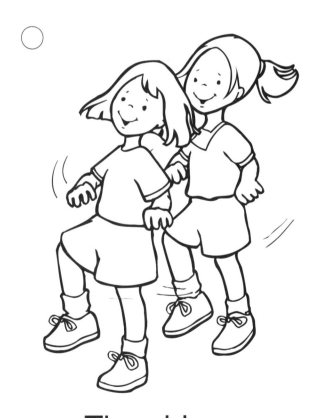

The girls are
skipping **forward**.

221

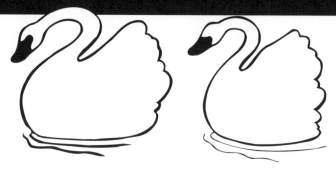

Concept: Forward

Date: _____

Ask your child to listen carefully as you read the following list of sentences slowly and clearly. It is important that your child not repeat the sentences but just listen to them quietly. Please spend one to two minutes daily reading these sentences to your child. After listening to these sentences, your child may color the pictures on the page!

1. The jets are flying forward.
2. The trucks are moving forward.
3. The elephants are dancing forward.
4. The monkeys are swinging forward.
5. The swans are swimming forward.
6. The marbles are rolling forward.
7. The turtles are walking forward.
8. The squirrels are looking forward.
9. The balls are bouncing forward.
10. The penguins are waddling forward.

Additional Comments/Helpful Hints:

_____

_____

_____

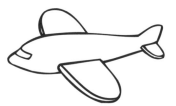

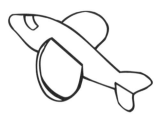

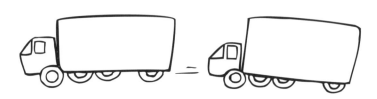

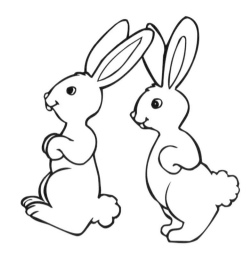

The rabbits are hopping **forward**.

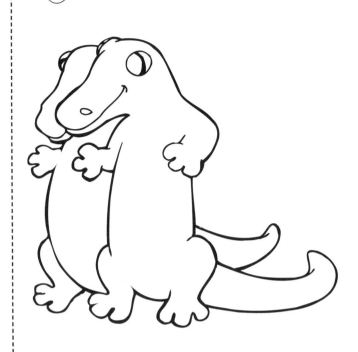

The alligators are walking **forward**.

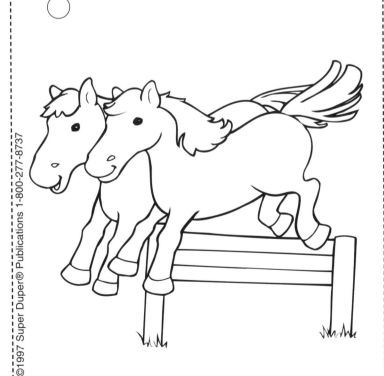

The horses are jumping **forward**.

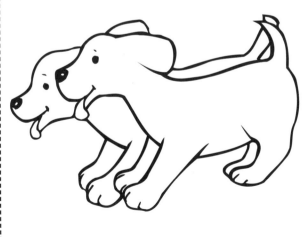

The dogs are running **forward**. 223

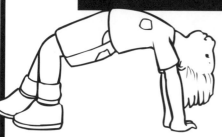
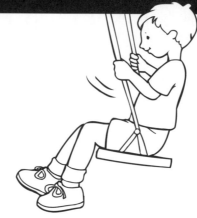
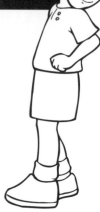

Home Speech Practice
Auditory Bombardment Sentences

Concept: Backward(s)*

Date: _____

Ask your child to listen carefully as you read the following list of sentences slowly and clearly. It is important that your child not repeat the sentences but just listen to them quietly. Please spend one to two minutes daily reading these sentences to your child. After listening to these sentences, your child may color the pictures on the page!

1. The boy is hopping backward(s).
2. The boy is looking backward(s).
3. The boy is diving backward(s).
4. The boy is bending backward(s).
5. The boy is jumping backward(s).
6. The boy is reaching backward(s).
7. The boy is swinging backward(s).
8. The boy is crawling backward(s).
9. The boy is walking backward(s).
10. The boy is kicking backward(s).

Additional Comments/Helpful Hints:

_____

_____

_____

* "Backward" or "Backwards" may be used interchangeably.

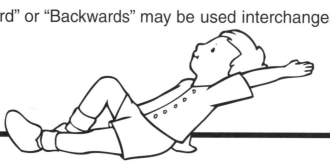
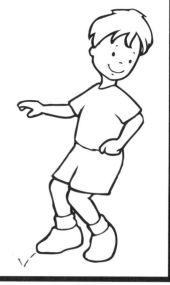

©1997 Super Duper® Publications 1-800-277-8737

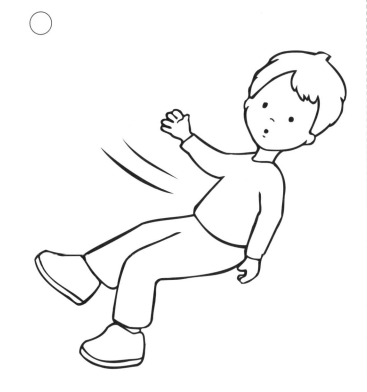

The boy is falling **backward(s)**.

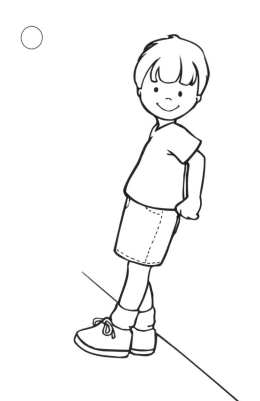

The boy is leaning **backward(s)**.

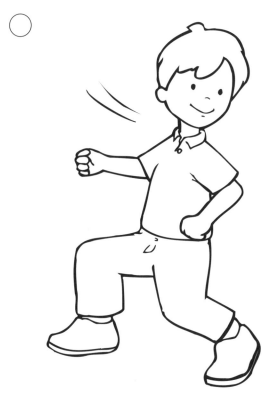

The boy is running **backward(s)**.

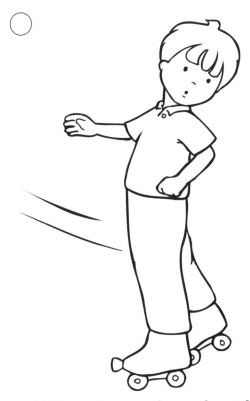

The boy is skating **backward(s)**.

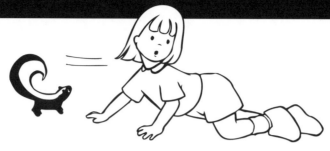

Home Speech Practice
Auditory Bombardment Sentences

Concept: Backward(s)*

Date: _____

Ask your child to listen carefully as you read the following list of sentences slowly and clearly. It is important that your child not repeat the sentences but just listen to them quietly. Please spend one to two minutes daily reading these sentences to your child. After listening to these sentences, your child may color the pictures on the page!

1. The girl is throwing backward(s).

2. The girl is hopping backward(s).

3. The girl is riding backward(s).

4. The girl is falling backward(s).

5. The girl is jogging backward(s).

6. The girl is skating backward(s).

7. The girl is jumping backward(s).

8. The girl is sliding backward(s).

9. The girl is crawling backward(s).

10. The girl is marching backward(s).

Additional Comments/Helpful Hints:

_____

_____

_____

* "Backward" or "Backwards" may be used interchangeably.

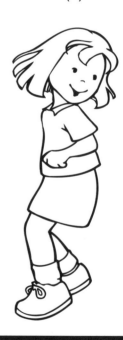

©1997 Super Duper® Publications 1-800-277-8737

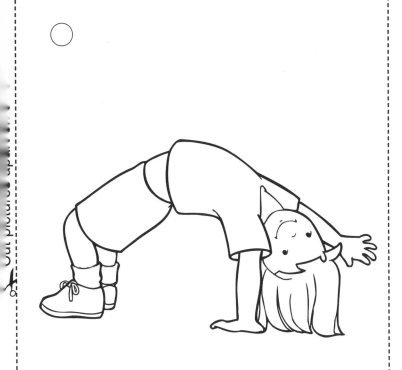

The girl is bending
backward(s).

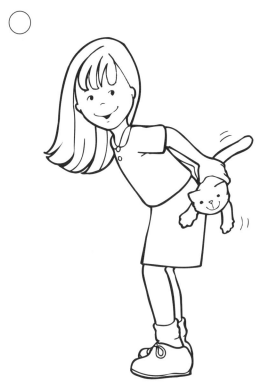

The girl is reaching
backward(s).

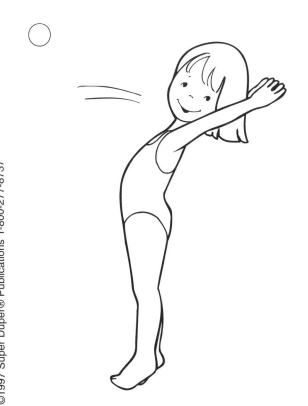

The girl is diving
backward(s).

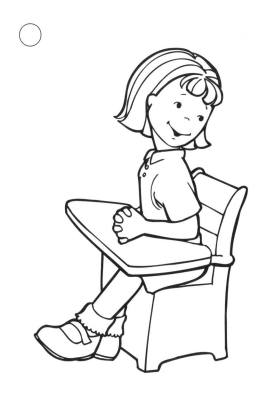

The girl is looking
backward(s).

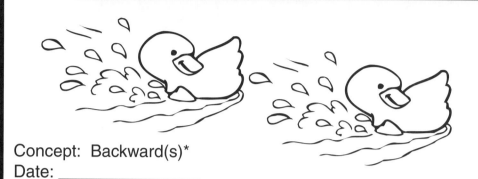
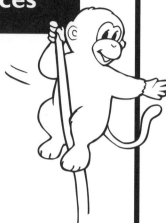

Concept: Backward(s)*

Date: _____

Ask your child to listen carefully as you read the following list of sentences slowly and clearly. It is important that your child not repeat the sentences but just listen to them quietly. Please spend one to two minutes daily reading these sentences to your child. After listening to these sentences, your child may color the pictures on the page!

1. The crab is crawling backward(s).

2. The monkey is reaching backward(s).

3. The cow is moving backward(s).

4. The donkey is kicking backward(s).

5. The dog is jumping backward(s).

6. The duck is swimming backward(s).

7. The seal is flipping backward(s).

8. The cat is creeping backward(s).

9. The tire is rolling backward(s).

10. The bear is falling backward(s).

Additional Comments/Helpful Hints:

_____

_____

_____

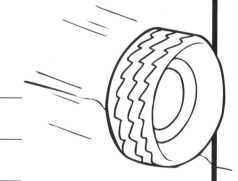

* "Backward" or "Backwards" may be used interchangeably.

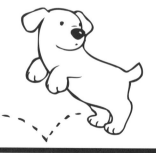

©1991 Super Duper® Publications 1-800-277-8737

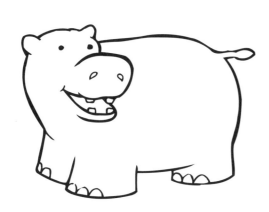

The hippopotamus is look-ing **backward(s)**.

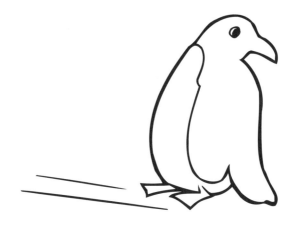

The penguin is sliding **backward(s)**.

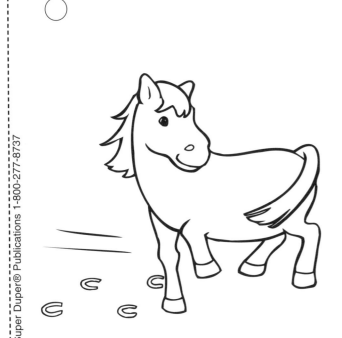

The horse is walking **backward(s)**.

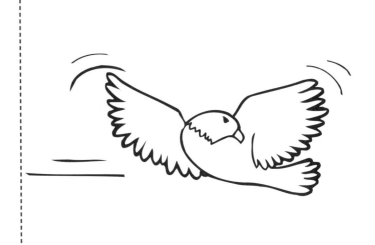

The eagle is flying **backward(s)**.

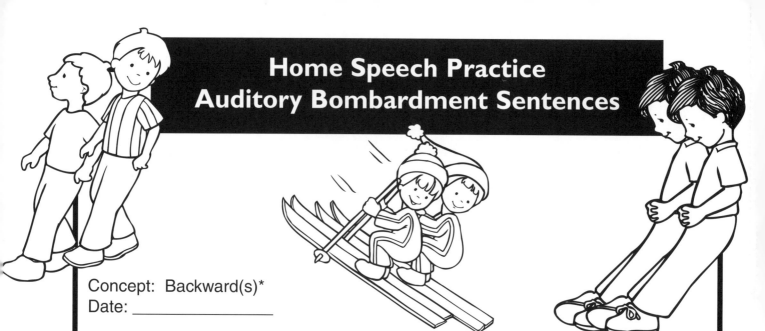

Home Speech Practice
Auditory Bombardment Sentences

Concept: Backward(s)*

Date: _____

Ask your child to listen carefully as you read the following list of sentences slowly and clearly. It is important that your child not repeat the sentences but just listen to them quietly. Please spend one to two minutes daily reading these sentences to your child. After listening to these sentences, your child may color the pictures on the page!

1. The boys are leaning backward(s).
2. The boys are bending backward(s).
3. The boys are swimming backward(s).
4. The boys are falling backward(s).
5. The boys are jumping backward(s).

6. The boys are dancing backward(s).
7. The boys are reaching backward(s).
8. The boys are skiing backward(s).
9. The boys are running backward(s).
10. The boys are walking backward(s).

Additional Comments/Helpful Hints:

_____

_____

_____

* "Backward" or "Backwards" may be used interchangeably.

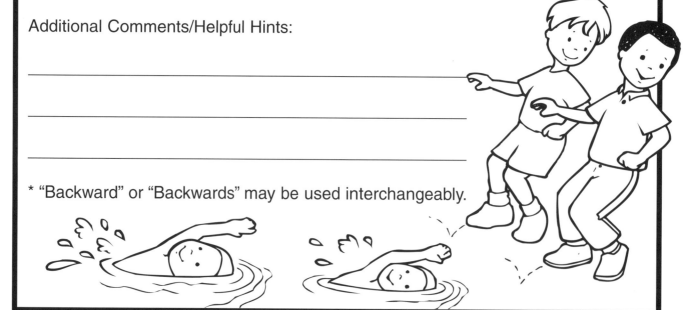

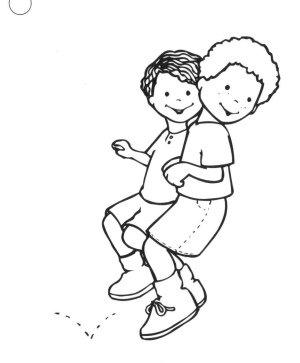

The boys are hopping **backward(s)**.

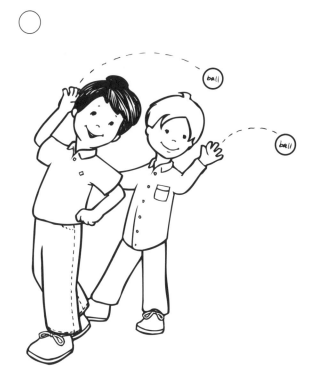

The boys are throwing **backward(s)**.

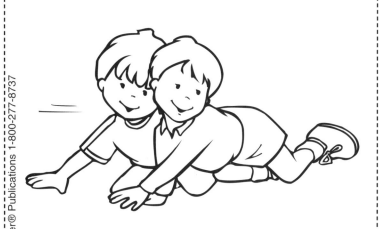

The boys are crawling **backward(s)**.

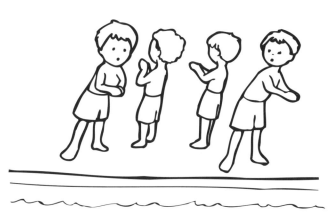

The boys are diving **backward(s)**.

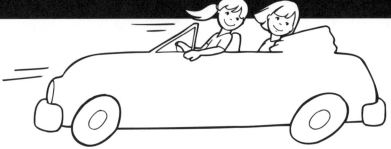

Home Speech Practice
Auditory Bombardment Sentences

Concept: Backwards

Date: _____

Ask your child to listen carefully as you read the following list of sentences slowly and clearly. It is important that your child not repeat the sentences but just listen to them quietly. Please spend one to two minutes daily reading these sentences to your child. After listening to these sentences, your child may color the pictures on the page!

1. The girls are skating backward(s).

2. The girls are walking backward(s).

3. The girls are moving backward(s).

4. The girls are looking backward(s).

5. The girls are swinging backward(s).

6. The girls are bending backward(s).

7. The girls are dancing backward(s).

8. The girls are diving backward(s).

9. The girls are hopping backward(s).

10. The girls are turning backward(s).

Additional Comments/Helpful Hints:

_____

_____

_____

* "Backward" or "Backwards" may be used interchangeably.

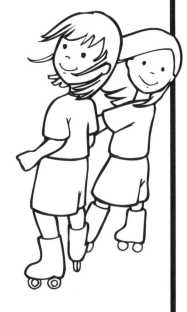

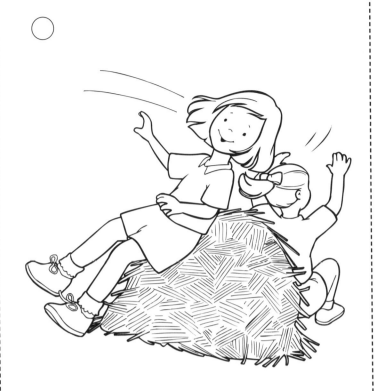

The girls are falling
backward(s).

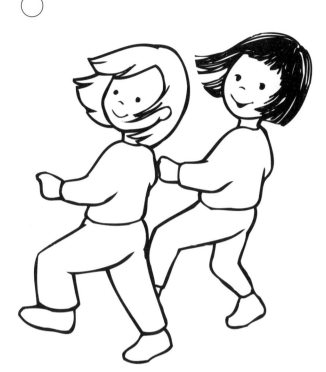

The girls are running
backward(s).

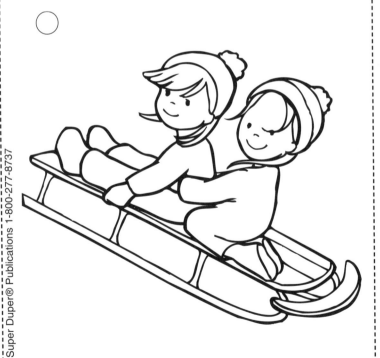

The girls are sliding
backward(s).

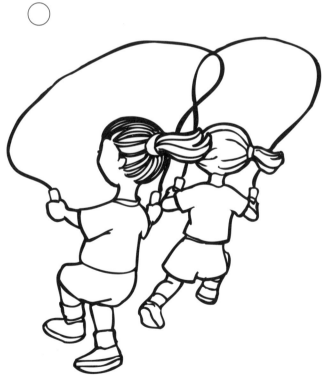

The girls are jumping
backward(s).

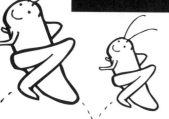

Home Speech Practice
Auditory Bombardment Sentences

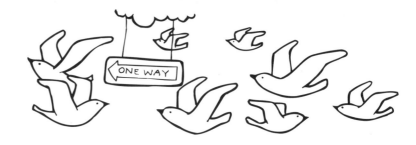

Concept: Backward(s)*

Date: _____

Ask your child to listen carefully as you read the following list of sentences slowly and clearly. It is important that your child not repeat the sentences but just listen to them quietly. Please spend one to two minutes daily reading these sentences to your child. After listening to these sentences, your child may color the pictures on the page!

1. The crickets are jumping backward(s).

2. The elephants are looking backward(s).

3. The geese are swimming backward(s).

4. The birds are flying backward(s).

5. The camels are moving backward(s).

6. The wheels are rolling backward(s).

7. The lobsters are crawling backward(s).

8. The balls are bouncing backward(s).

9. The horses are walking backward(s).

10. The seals are sliding backward(s).

Additional Comments/Helpful Hints:

_____

_____

_____

* "Backward" or "Backwards" may be used interchangeably.

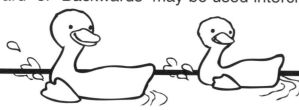

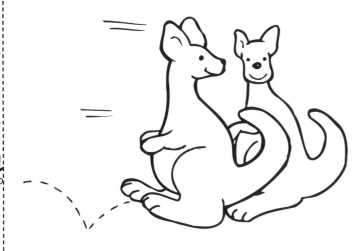

The kangaroos are
hopping **backward(s)**.

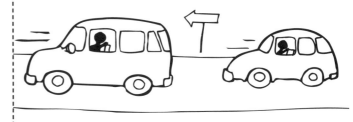

The cars are going
backward(s).

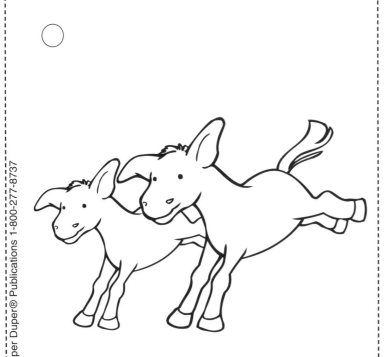

The donkeys are
kicking **backward(s)**.

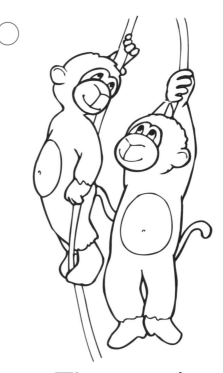

The monkeys
are swinging
backward(s).

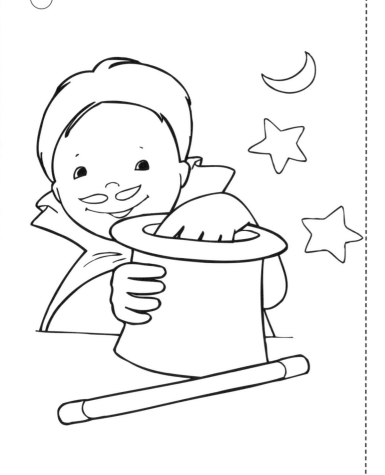

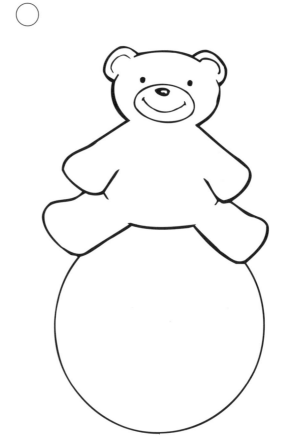

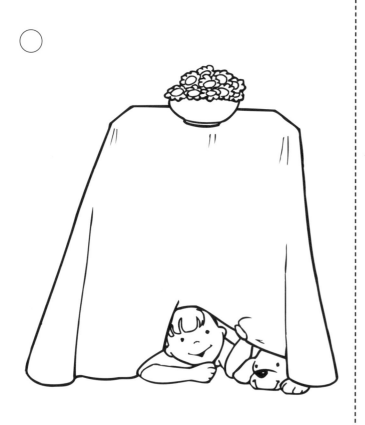

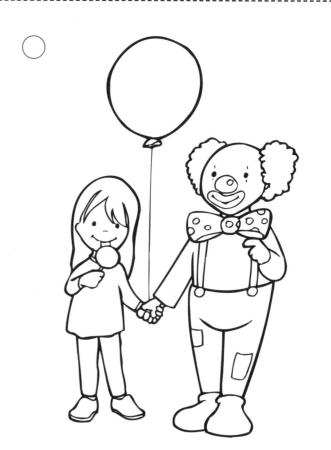

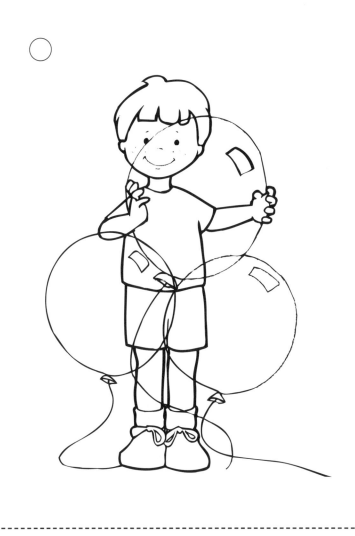

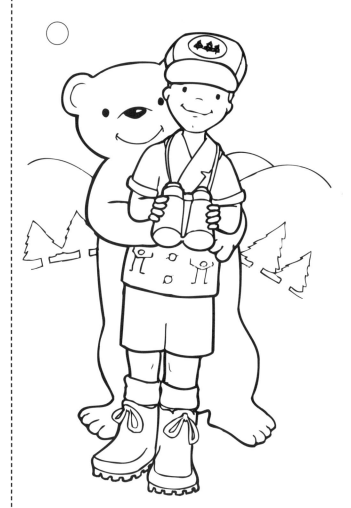

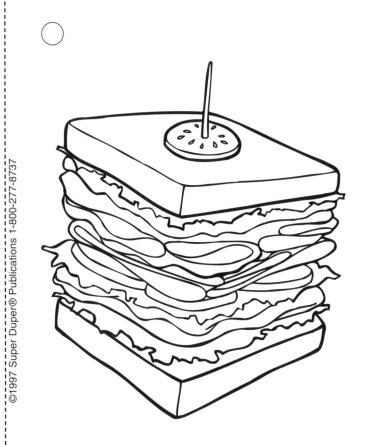

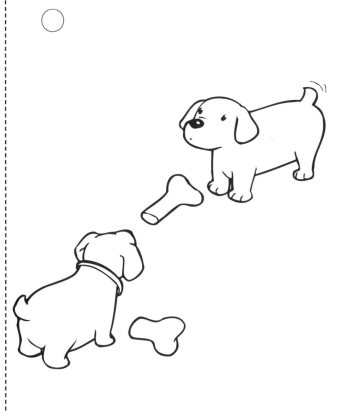

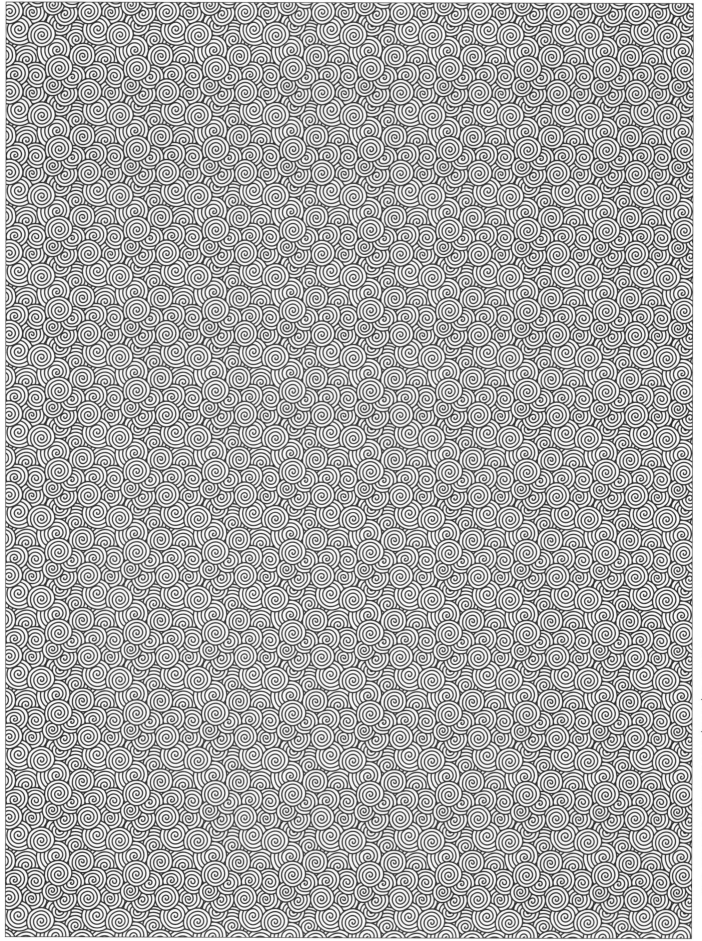

238

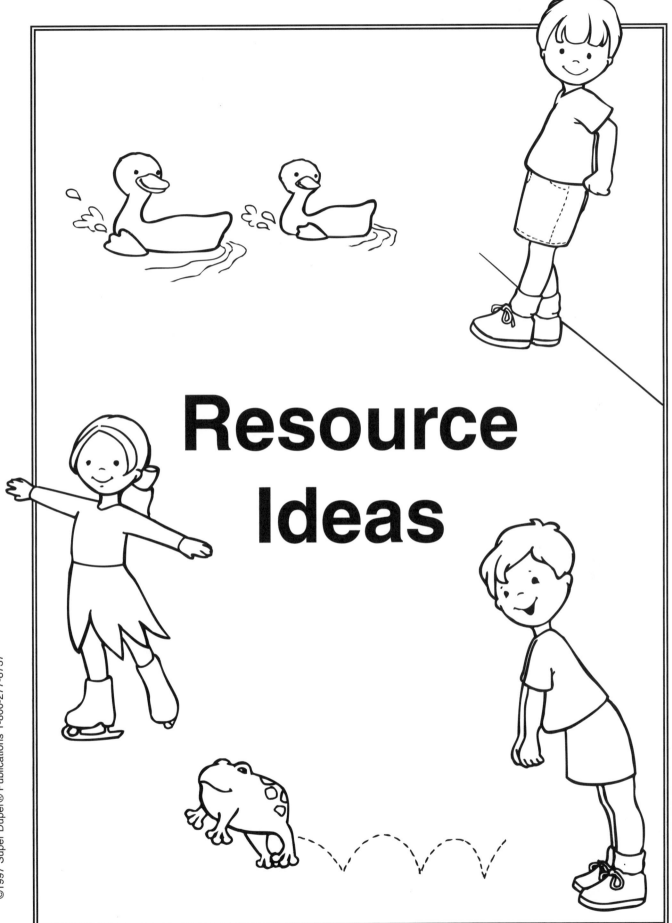

Resource Ideas

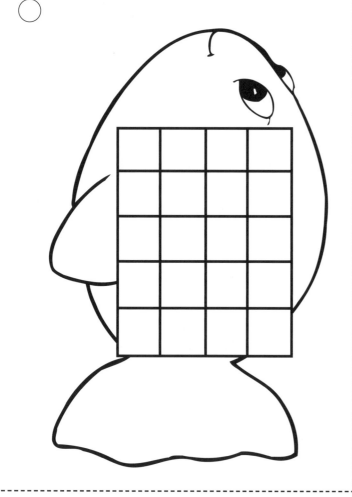

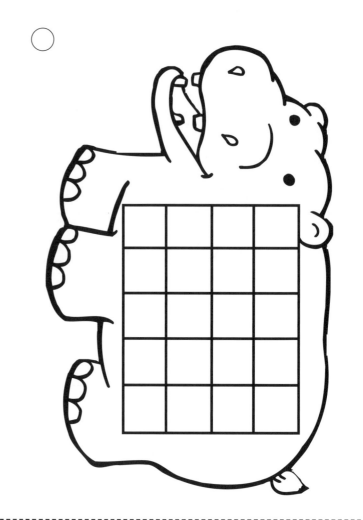

cut pictures apart on dotted line

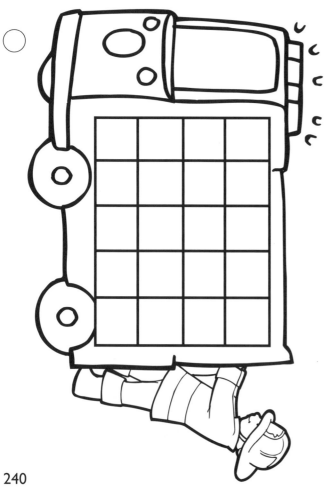

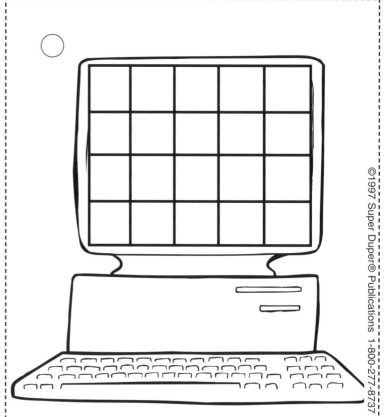

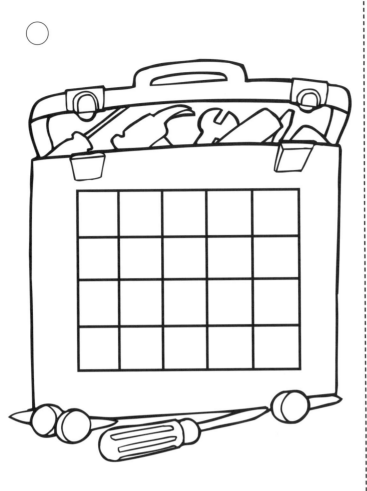

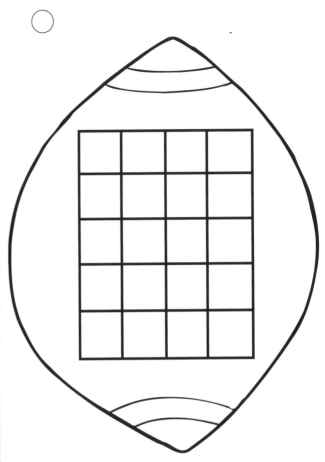

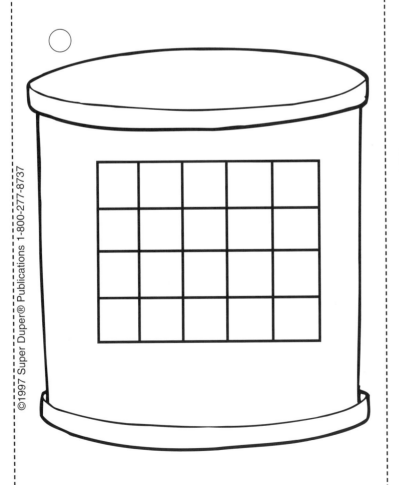

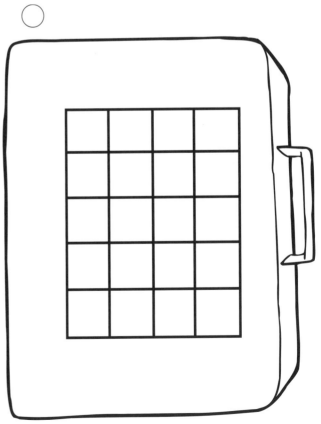

241

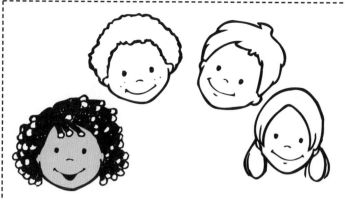

In speech today,
I learned four _____.
Ask me to name them!

No Lion! I can name a few
_____.
Try me!

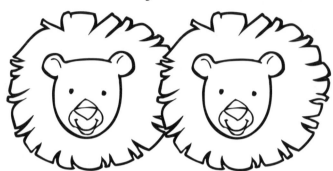

Now I know four new
_____.
Just ask me!

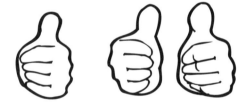

Wow! Ask me to name four
_____.
Bet I can!

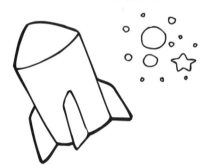

I worked very hard in speech
today! Let me name four
_____ for you!

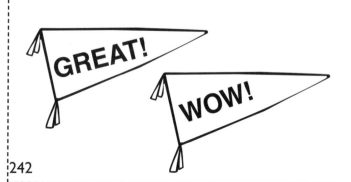

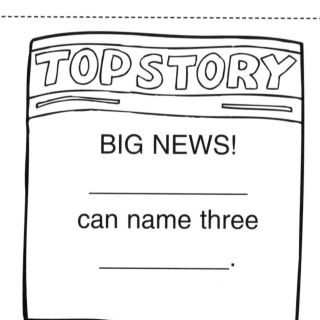

TOP STORY

BIG NEWS!

_____
can name three
_____.

A "Two Thumbs" up performance in speech today! BRAVO!

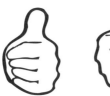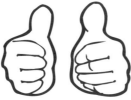

BREAKING NEWS! _____ worked very hard in speech today. Thought you should know!

4

Flew in to tell you _____

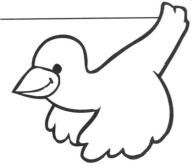

had a fantastic day in speech! Keep up the good work!

Super Speech Star!

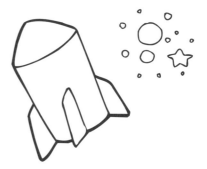

_____

_____ was a terrific helper in speech today!

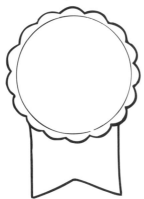

Doggone good behavior in speech today!

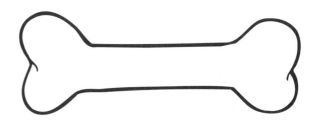

Extra! Extra! Read All About It!

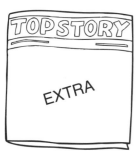

_____

has successfully
completed the language
program at

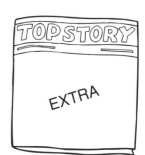

_____.

Proudly Presented By _____
Date _____

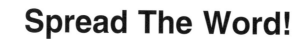

Spread The Word!

_____

has completed the vocabulary program at

_____.

_____
Speech-Language Pathologist

_____
Date

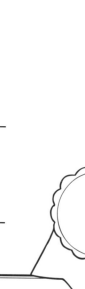

Certificate of Completion

_____ has completed the

language program at _____.

Congratulations!

Presented by _____

Date _____

#1   **Language Diploma**   **#1**

This diploma hereby certifies that
_____ has successfully
completed the language program at
_____.

This diploma is proudly presented by
_____ on _____.

Speech-Language Pathologist

Egg-cellent Work!

_____

has completed the vocabulary
program at

_____

_____
Speech-Language Pathologist

_____
Date

LOOKING GOOD!

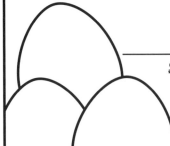
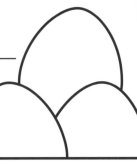

_____

HAS COMPLETED THE LANGUAGE
PROGRAM AT

_____

_____
SPEECH-LANGUAGE PATHOLOGIST

_____
DATE

Certificate of Completion

_____

has completed the vocabulary program at

_____ .

Congratulations!

Presented by _____

Speech-Language Pathologist

on _____ .

Date

 # LANGUAGE STAR!

_____

HAS COMPLETED THE LANGUAGE PROGRAM AT

_____ .

_____

SPEECH-LANGUAGE PATHOLOGIST

_____

DATE

ADDITIONAL IDEAS FOR THERAPY

1. **Treasure Hunt -** The student tries to find hidden pictures or objects in the classroom. When the object/picture is found, the student names it or uses the word in a sentence.

2. **Puzzle Mania -** The student is given one piece of puzzle for every correct response. Once the pieces have been collected, the student can put the puzzle together.

3. **Buried Treasure -** Pictures or objects are buried in a box of rice, sand, beans, etc. The student finds the target picture/object and then names it.

4. **Jump Rope Frenzy -** The student jumps rope while producing the target word with every jump.

5. **Fishing Game -** Make a fishing pole using a small wooden dowel with a string attached. (The string should be approximately 16 to 18 inches.) At the end of the string, place a magnet. (The horseshoe-shaped magnets work the best.) To each target picture, attach a paper clip. Now the student can fish for the target words by dropping the magnet at the end of the fishing pole to "catch" a target picture.

6. **Clothespin Drop -** The student can kneel on a chair (or stand) and drop clothespins into a jar below. With each drop, the student will verbalize the target word.

7. **Fruit Loop/Cheerios Paste-up -** The student will glue Fruit Loops® or Cheerios® to a target vocabulary word or picture on tagboard.

8. **HopScotch -** The clinician makes a hopscotch outline using chalk or masking tape. One target picture is placed on each square of the hop-scotch outline. The student names the target picture prior to hopping to the next square.

9. **Guessing Game -** The clinician tapes a target word on the student's back. The student must guess the unknown picture by asking yes/no questions to the clinician or other students.

10. **Hidden Pictures -** Objects or target pictures are hidden around the room. The clinician turns off the lights and gives the student a flashlight to hunt for them. The student names each picture/object as it is found.

11. **Hot Potato -** Two target pictures are taped to a beanbag hot potato or a real potato. As the potato is tossed, the student names the target picture.

12. **Stopwatch Race -** The student names as many target pictures as possible in one minute.

13. **Play Dough Sculptures -** The student reproduces the target pictures using play dough.

14. **Building Blocks -** The student receives one block for every correct response. He/She can build towers, houses, buildings, etc.

15. **Bowling Bonanza -** The clinician tapes target words on toy bowling pins. The student tries to knock down as many pins as he/she can with the bowling ball. The student then names all the target pictures on the pins that were knocked down.

©1997 Super Duper® Publications 1-800-277-8737

16. **Memory Game** - The clinician chooses four or more target pictures. The student then looks at the pictures for 30 seconds. The student is asked to close his/her eyes as the clinician turns one picture over. The student opens his/her eyes and has to guess which picture has been turned over.

17. **Feely Box or Grab Bag** - The clinician fills a box or bag with objects/pictures containing target vocabulary words. The student then pulls out each object/picture and names it.

18. **Bean Bag Toss** - The student will throw a bean bag through a standing figure with holes in it. (The figure can be a clown, cowboy, etc.) Above each hole, a target picture can be taped. When the student throws a bean bag through a hole, he/she names the target picture.

19. **Vocabulary Charades** - The student acts out a target vocabulary word such as "chef," "mow," "snake," etc. Other students take turns guessing the target word.

20. **Listen "Beary" Carefully** - The student listens and corrects a word in a sentence. For example, with animal vocabulary words:

    I like the nursery rhyme, "Three Blind R-ice. (mice)"
    An animal that barks is a h-og. (dog)
    Do you like the story "Goldilocks and the Three H-airs? (bears)"

©1997 Super Duper® Publications 1-800-277-8737

Notes

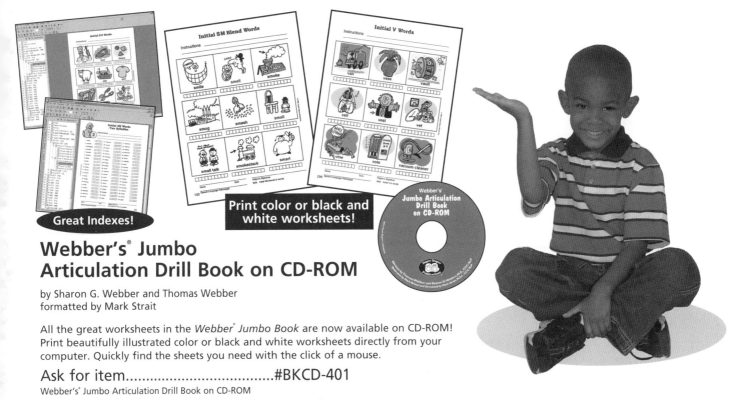

Webber's® Jumbo
Articulation Drill Book on CD-ROM

by Sharon G. Webber and Thomas Webber
formatted by Mark Strait

All the great worksheets in the *Webber Jumbo Book* are now available on CD-ROM! Print beautifully illustrated color or black and white worksheets directly from your computer. Quickly find the sheets you need with the click of a mouse.

Ask for item....................................#BKCD-401
Webber's® Jumbo Articulation Drill Book on CD-ROM

Ask for item....................................#BKCD-402
Webber's® Jumbo Artic Combo

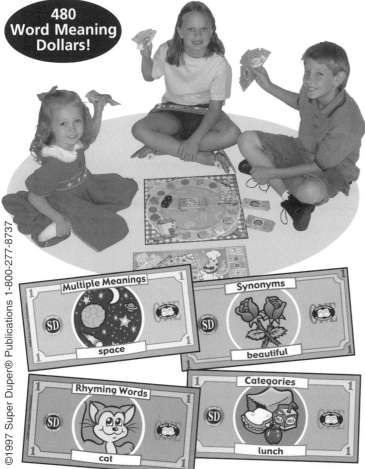

480 Word Meaning Dollars!

Go for the Dough!® Board Game
The Game of Word Meanings and More!

Grades PreK and Up

by Margaret Froitzheim and Clint Johnson

Deliver pizzas, make big bucks, and increase word meaning vocabulary! This fast-paced, vocabulary enriching, word meaning (semantics) board game will help your children improve their word recall, describing, semantic flexibility, and phonemic awareness skills.

Players start at the Pizza Palace. As students drive their cars around the board to deliver their imaginary pizzas, they choose Super Dough Dollars™. Each Dollar targets Categories, Definitions, Multiple Meanings, Opposites, Rhyming Words, or Synonyms. (You choose one category before the game begins, or mix and match!) Students provide a word or definition based on the language objective, and place the Dollars in the center of the board. Each time a player reaches Grandma's house to deliver a "pizza," he/she gets "paid" with all the Dollars on the board!

Each of the 480 Super Dough Dollars™ reviews a language skill that is crucial in expanding word knowledge. Best of all, the Dollars feel like real money - and won't tear or rip!

Go for the Dough!® targets:

* 80 Synonyms.
* 80 Opposites.
* 80 Rhyming Words.
* 80 Categories.
* 80 Multiple Meanings.
* 80 Definitions.

It includes a colorful, sturdy 16″ x 16″ game board, 480 Super Dough Dollars™ (4½″ x 2⅛″), six car pawns, a die, and a booklet containing suggested answers. Any way you slice it, there's no "topping" *Go for the Dough!®*

Ask for item.............................#GB-339
Go for the Dough!®

Descripto™ Dinos Vocabulary Game Boards

14 Games

Grades PreK-5

By Melissa Bossert, Kimberly Marino, Sharon G. Webber & Nancy Fulton

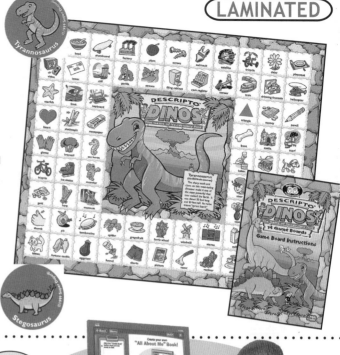

Your students' describing skills will take giant leaps with these jumbo 15″ x 18″ *Descripto™ Dinos Game Boards*. To play, students place a Dino token on a vocabulary picture and roll the die. The number on the spinner determines how many "descriptions" the student must say about the picture. For example, if the player chooses the apple picture and the spinner lands on the number four, the student would tell four things about an apple. (It is red, has a stem, grows on a tree, and is a fruit.) Each game can be customized based on the level of each student. Great for vocabulary building too! Descripto™ Dinos includes:

- 14 colorful, laminated games (7 boards printed front and back).

- Each board contains 74 vocabulary picture words, for a total of 1,036 picture words!

- A die and instruction book!

- 90 roaringly bright dino tokens in assorted colors!

Ask for Item.................#DD-12
Descripto™ Dinos Game Boards

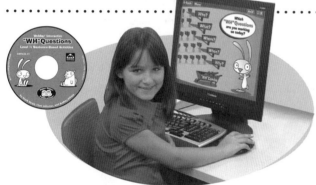

Webber® Interactive "WH" Questions CD-ROM

Level 1: Sentence-Based Activities

Grades PreK and Up

by Mark Strait, Clint Johnson, Audrey Prince & Tawnia Lechner

Webber® Interactive "WH" Questions Level 1: Sentence-Based Activities helps students practice and learn how to ask and answer WH questions (Who, What, Where, When, and Why). It has 375 questions/answers divided into four sections:

- Learn About WH Questions reviews the types of WH Questions and presents color-coded symbols to help students remember them.

- Answer Simple WH Questions provides practice answering simple WH questions.

- Choose the Correct WH Questions provides practice matching an answer to the correct WH question.

- Answer WH Inference Questions provides practice using a picture to infer the answer to a WH question.

Webber® Interactive "WH" Questions also allows the teacher to track and collect data for an unlimited number of students and increases the difficulty level by changing the program settings.

Ask for Item...............................#WHCD-11
Webber® Interactive "WH" Questions Level 1

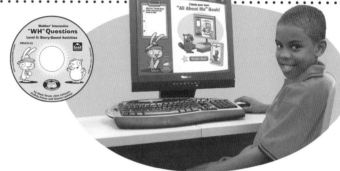

Webber® Interactive "WH" Questions CD-ROM

Level 2: Story-Based Activities

Grades PreK and Up

by Mark Strait, Clint Johnson, Audrey Prince & Tawnia Lechner

Webber® Interactive "WH" Questions Level 2: Story-Based Activities helps students practice and learn how to ask and answer WH Questions (Who, What, Where, When, and Why) in stories and to answer personal WH questions as they create their own book about themselves. It has four activities:

- Learn About WH Questions is a short tutorial that reviews the five types of WH questions.

- Answer WH Questions in Stories provides practice listening to 25 short stories and answering WH questions that have <u>two</u> answer choices.

- Build a Story provides practice listening to the same 25 stories and answering WH questions that have <u>five</u> answer choices.

- Answering Personal WH Questions ("All About Me" Book) lets the student create his/her own book by answering personal WH questions that relate directly to the student.

Webber® Interactive "WH" Questions also allows the teacher to track and collect data for an unlimited number of students and increase difficulty levels by changing the program settings.

Ask for Item...............................#WHCD-22
Webber® Interactive "WH" Questions Level 2

©1997 Super Duper® Publications 1-800-277-8737

Call 1-800-277-8737
FAX 1-800-978-7379

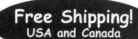
Free Shipping!
USA and Canada

www.superduperinc.com
Order Anytime!